# THE WHITEBOARD DAILY BOOK OF CUES FOR EVERYONE

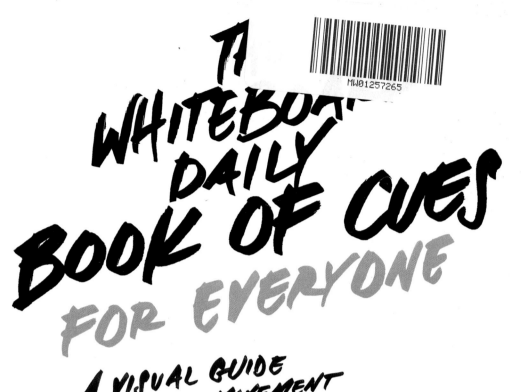

## A VISUAL GUIDE TO EFFICIENT MOVEMENT FOR ANY FITNESS LEVEL, AGE, AND DISCIPLINE

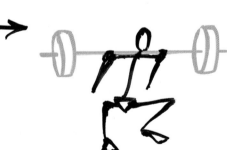

## KARL EAGLEMAN

VICTORY BELT PUBLISHING INC.

LAS VEGAS

*This book is dedicated to my students, the Olympians of Columbus East High School.*

## ACKNOWLEDGMENTS

**To my wife, Ali:** *Thank you for always being supportive and encouraging of this passion project of mine. Thank you for being my partner with this and in life.*

**To Charlotte Kughen, Susan Lloyd, and Lance Freimuth:** *If it weren't for you, this book and the previous one would not have been a reality. No question. Thank you for believing in me, your hard work, and your expertise to make this project successful.*

**To Columbus East High School:** *Thank you for blessing me with the opportunity and support to coach hundreds of athletes every year. At the end of each day, I have never been so exhausted yet more fulfilled.*

First published in 2024 by Victory Belt Publishing Inc.

Copyright © 2024 Karl Eagleman

ISBN-13: 978-1-628605-56-3

Cover design by Karl Eagleman and Kat Lannom

Interior design by Yordan Terziev and Boryana Yordanova

Illustrations by Karl Eagleman

Printed in Canada

TC 0124

# CONTENTS

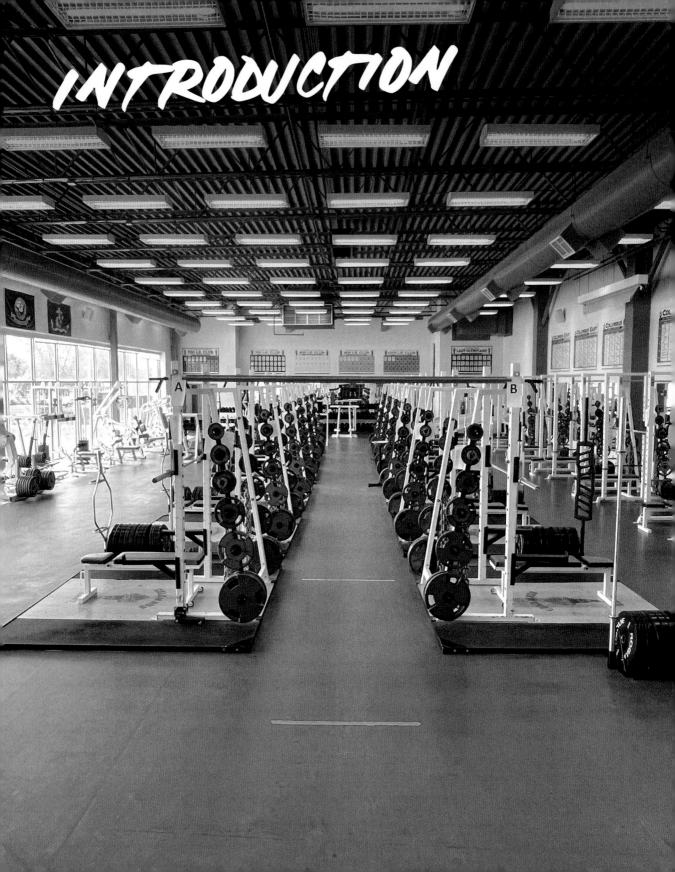

# INTRODUCTION

They say that if you want to learn to speak French, move to France. That's a way of saying that if you want to learn to do something well, you should immerse yourself in it. Surround yourself with the subject matter. Allow it to become a way of life.

For the past three years, I've had the privilege of serving as the head strength and conditioning coach for Columbus East High School in Columbus, Indiana. Two hundred forty students participate in my eighty-eight-minute weight training classes. Following my last class of the day, I oversee a program called East Beast, where I lead our off-season athletes through their after-school weight training.

Throughout the week, I walk an average eight miles a day as I go up and down the aisles between our eighteen lifting platforms, watch students move, and guide them to be more efficient. I'm completely immersed in watching, assessing, and coaching movement. In other words, I moved to France.

The language I study is movement. Rather than studying subjects and predicates, my focus is the agreement between stance, grip, and position. I study how ankles, knees, hips, and shoulders move in relation to each other. Then I communicate feedback to thirteen- to eighteen-year-olds in a way they can clearly understand and implement.

At the end of each day, I am completely exhausted but also equally fulfilled. I truly feel that I am helping athletes become stronger versions of themselves, and I hope I'm leading them to understand that hard work pays off.

Throughout each day, I gather inspiration from the cues I give to my students so I can illustrate them to share on Whiteboard Daily. I figure if some perspective or analogy helped me communicate movement to an athlete, other coaches and athletes may find it helpful.

I've also discovered that if you want to understand something better, you should try drawing it. Even if you have zero artistic ability, when you attempt to illustrate a thought or idea, you're forced to understand the details of the subject. For example, how do you explain where the knees are relative to the ankles during a movement sequence? Where are the hips relative to the shoulders? These little details make a big difference, and figuring out how to draw them has helped me become a much better coach.

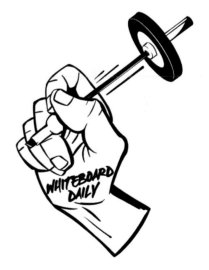

To excel as an effective coach, you must be passionate about learning. When you stop learning, you stop growing, and your athletes will notice. Just as you strive to have your athletes achieve virtuosity within their movement, hold the same standard for yourself and your coaching.

The individuals I coach have different levels of skill, strength, and ability. Serving such a diverse population means that to communicate movement successfully, I need a good-sized coaching toolbox to hold the collection of cues and methods I've acquired over the years. Now, I've compiled that knowledge into this book (and my first book, *The Whiteboard Daily Book of Cues*) so you can add these cues to your toolbox as well.

Whether you're a coach, an athlete, or someone who just wants to improve their own movement, I'm certain that within this book you will find many cues that will help you understand and communicate movement in new ways.

# HOW TO USE THIS BOOK AND THE CUES

In this book, the whiteboards are categorized as Coaching Cues, Education, Perspective, Skill Transfer, Movement Library, Coaching Education, and Coaching Perspective. The information on each whiteboard should be helpful regardless of whether you're a coach who's trying to help others or an athlete who's trying to improve on your own. And when it comes to the Coaching Education and Coaching Perspective tidbits, you may even find that they're applicable to your life outside of the gym.

Every good coach learns from other coaches, and by no means are all of the cues in this book my original ideas. You'll find a lot of hat tips (h/t) throughout the book, and I encourage you to check out the work of those coaches as well!

## WHAT IS A CUE?

Cues are directions to improve movement. They give a body part a direction: "chest up," "knees out," "flex your butt." They should be specific, actionable, and short. This makes them easier to remember and quickly applicable.

Cues fall into four primary categories:

- **Verbal cues:** Using your voice to communicate movement—"JUMP!"
- **Visual cues:** Using your body to demonstrate movement—standing in front of your athlete and performing an air squat.
- **Mental cues:** Using imagery to describe movement—"Imagine you are screwing your feet into the ground."
- **Tactile cues:** Using touch or physical feedback to communicate what the athlete needs to do—squatting to a box.

# A FEW THINGS TO CONSIDER

**There is no such thing as a "golden cue."** No cue works for every person every time. Since all athletes are unique and learn in different ways, it's important to have a variety of cues to address an issue. A larger mental toolbox gives you the potential to be an even better coach.

**Give one cue at a time.** When you watch a novice athlete move, they will likely display a number of movement inefficiencies. Rather than providing the athlete with a laundry list of items to fix, focus on the one that addresses their safety first and then triage from there. Hint: Work from the ground up when it comes to fixing movement. Most issues start with balance in the feet.

**Cues should address the positive, not the negative.** Saying, "Don't lower your elbows," doesn't provide specific instruction. The athlete may think, *Okay, then where* do *I put my elbows?* Tell the athlete what they *should do,* not the opposite.

**Demonstrate the cue when you deliver it.** Just as some people "talk with their hands," you should use your body to show what you mean when you say the cue.

**Avoid using the same cue over and over again.** If you do not see an improvement in the athlete's movement after you have provided a cue, try using a different cue or a combination of cues—e.g., tactile cue + verbal cue.

**Know *when* to introduce a new cue.** Warm-ups and working sets are the perfect time to deliver a new cue. This will be during a time when the athlete is fresh and the weight is manageable. Never introduce a new cue when the athlete is attempting to lift a weight that is more than 80 percent of their one-rep max (1RM). During that time, it is important for the athlete to focus on familiar concepts that have proven to work for them.

Get creative! Maya Angelou said, "You can't use up creativity. The more you use, the more you have." The same applies to communicating movement. The exercises we do in the gym are supposed to make us stronger for our activity in the real world. Use that connection to make movement relatable.

# CHAPTER ①

# FOUNDATIONAL MOVEMENTS

# AIR SQUAT

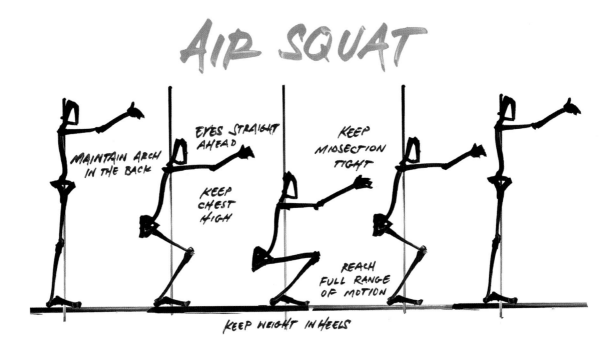

MAINTAIN ARCH IN THE BACK

EYES STRAIGHT AHEAD

KEEP CHEST HIGH

KEEP MIDSECTION TIGHT

REACH FULL RANGE OF MOTION

KEEP WEIGHT IN HEELS

## Points of Performance

**Setup:**

Stance that allows full range of motion below parallel

**Movement:**

- Keep your trunk and neck in a neutral position.
- Keep weight in the tripod of your foot (first toe, pinky toe, heel).
- Keep your chest high.
- Keep your knees in line with your toes.
- Reach the full range of motion (below parallel).

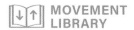
# BACK SQUAT

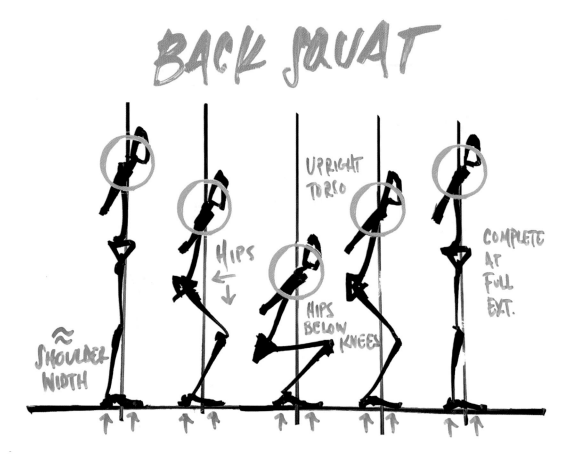

## Points of Performance

### Setup:

- Approximate shoulder-width stance
- Hands just outside shoulders with full grip on the bar
- Bar resting on your shoulders
- Elbows pointed down and behind bar

### Movement:

- Your hips descend back and down and go lower than your knees.
- Maintain your spine's lumbar curve.
- Keep your heels grounded.
- Your knees are in line with your toes' direction.
- The movement is complete at full hip and knee extension.

# THE FRONT SQUAT

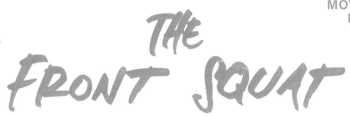

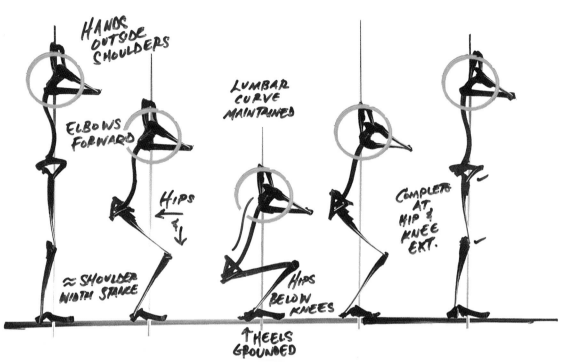

HANDS OUTSIDE SHOULDERS

ELBOWS FORWARD

LUMBAR CURVE MAINTAINED

HIPS &

≈ SHOULDER WIDTH STANCE

HIPS BELOW KNEES

↑HEELS GROUNDED

COMPLETE AT HIP & KNEE EXT.

## Points of Performance

**Setup:**

- Stance that allows full range of motion below parallel
- Loose fingertip grip on the bar
- Grip width is outside of shoulders
- Elbows point forward

**Movement:**

- Keep your trunk and neck in a neutral position.
- Keep weight in the tripod of your foot (first toe, pinky toe, heel).
- Keep your chest high.
- Knees in line with your toes.
- Reach the full range of motion (below parallel).

# THE OVERHEAD SQUAT

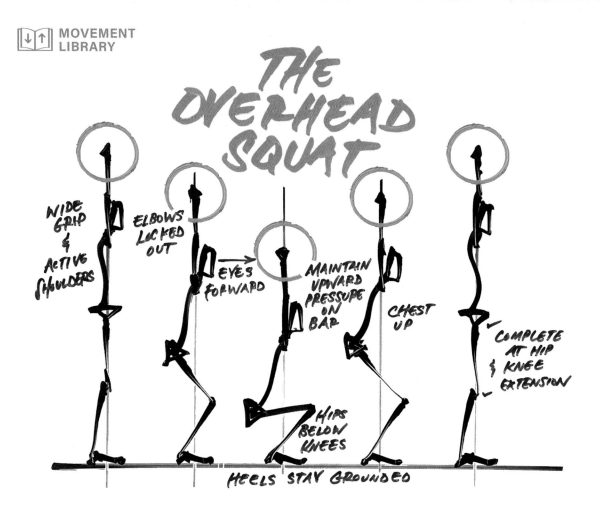

WIDE GRIP & ACTIVE SHOULDERS

ELBOWS LOCKED OUT

EYES FORWARD

MAINTAIN UPWARD PRESSURE ON BAR

CHEST UP

COMPLETE AT HIP & KNEE EXTENSION

HIPS BELOW KNEES

HEELS STAY GROUNDED

## Points of Performance

**Setup:**

- Stance that allows full range of motion below parallel

- Wide grip on the bar

- Active shoulders (elbows pointed down, armpits pointing forward)

- Elbows locked out

**Movement:**

- Keep your trunk and neck in a neutral position.

- Bar stays over the middle of your foot.

- Keep weight in the tripod of your foot.

- Keep your chest high.

- Knees in line with your toes.

- Reach the full range of motion (below parallel).

The movement is complete at full knee and hip extension with the bar over the center of your foot.

# THE STRICT PRESS
## AKA. SHOULDER PRESS

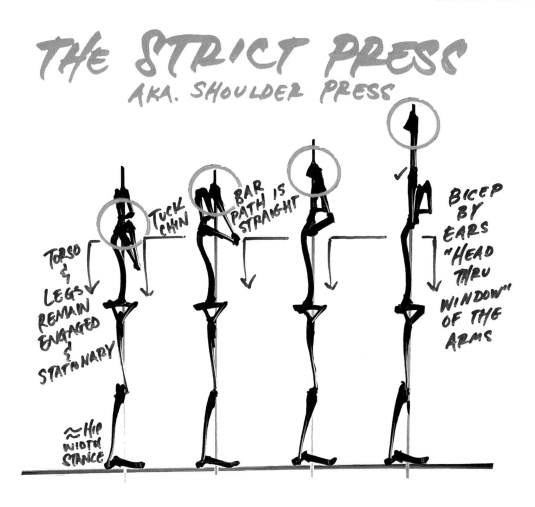

TORSO & LEGS REMAIN ENGAGED & STATIONARY

TUCK CHIN

BAR PATH IS STRAIGHT

BICEP BY EARS "HEAD THRU WINDOW" OF THE ARMS

≈ HIP WIDTH STANCE

## Points of Performance

### Setup:

- Hip-width stance
- Grip width just outside of shoulders
- Elbows slightly in front of the bar
- Full grip on the bar
- Bar rests on the torso

### Movement:

- Keep your torso and lower body stationary and engaged.
- Keep the bar in line over the middle of your foot.
- Complete at full arm, hip, and knee extension.

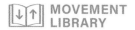

# THE PUSH PRESS

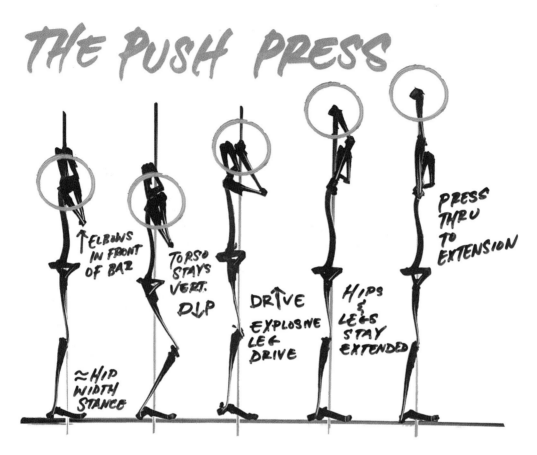

ELBOWS IN FRONT OF BAR

↑ HIP WIDTH STANCE

TORSO STAYS VERT. DIP

DRIVE EXPLOSIVE LEG DRIVE

HIPS & LEGS STAY EXTENDED

PRESS THRU TO EXTENSION

## Points of Performance

**Setup:**

- Hip-width stance
- Grip width just outside of shoulders
- Elbows slightly in front of the bar
- Full grip on the bar
- Bar rests on the torso

**Movement:**

- Dip your torso straight down.
- Rapidly extend your hips and legs and then press.
- Keep your heels down until you extend your hips and legs.
- Keep the bar in line over the middle of your foot.
- Complete at full arm, hip, and knee extension.

# THE PUSH JERK

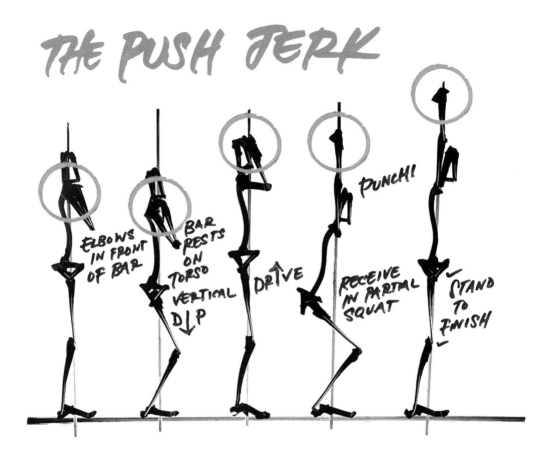

ELBOWS IN FRONT OF BAR

BAR RESTS ON TORSO

VERTICAL DIP

DRIVE

PUNCH!

RECEIVE IN PARTIAL SQUAT

STAND TO FINISH

## Points of Performance

### Setup:

- Hip-width stance
- Grip width just outside of shoulders
- Elbows slightly in front of the bar
- Full grip on the bar

### Movement:

- Dip your torso straight down.
- Rapidly extend your hips and legs and then press under.
- Keep your heels down until your hips and legs fully extend.
- Receive the bar in a partial overhead position.
- Keep the bar in line over the middle of your foot.
- Complete at full arm, hip, and knee extension.

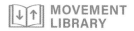
# THE DEADLIFT

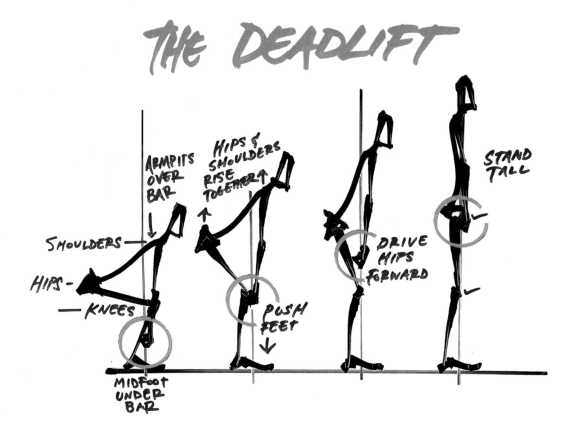

ARMPITS OVER BAR

HIPS & SHOULDERS RISE TOGETHER

STAND TALL

SHOULDERS —

HIPS —

— KNEES

PUSH FEET

DRIVE HIPS FORWARD

MIDFOOT UNDER BAR

## Points of Performance

### Setup:

- Hip-width stance
- Grip width just outside of shoulders
- Elbows slightly in front of the bar
- Full grip on the bar
- Bar rests on the torso

### Movement:

- Maintain lumbar curve.
- Bring up hips and shoulders at the same rate.
- Keep the bar in line over the middle of your foot.
- Keep your heels down.
- Complete at full hip and knee extension.

# "SUMO DEADLIFT HIGH PULL"

- WIDE STANCE
- NARROW GRIP
- KNEES TRACK OVER TOES

EXTEND HIPS ⟶ SHRUG ⟶ ELBOWS PULL HIGH & TO REAR

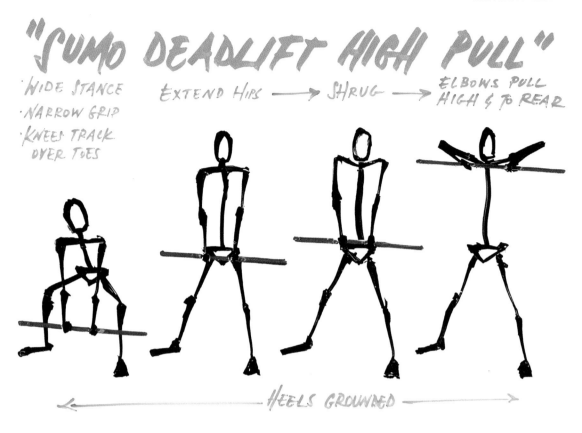

← ——— HEELS GROUNDED ——— →

## Points of Performance

### Setup:

- Stance slightly wider than shoulder width
- Grip width inside knees
- Full grip on bar
- Shoulders start slightly in front of bar

### Movement:

- Bring up hips and shoulders at the same rate; then extend hips.
- Shrug your shoulders and then move elbows high and behind.
- Keep the bar in line over the middle of your foot.
- Keep your trunk and neck in a neutral position.
- Keep your weight in the tripod of your foot (first toe, pinky toe, heel).
- Complete at full hip and knee extension with bar under chin.

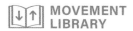
# THE MEDICINE BALL CLEAN

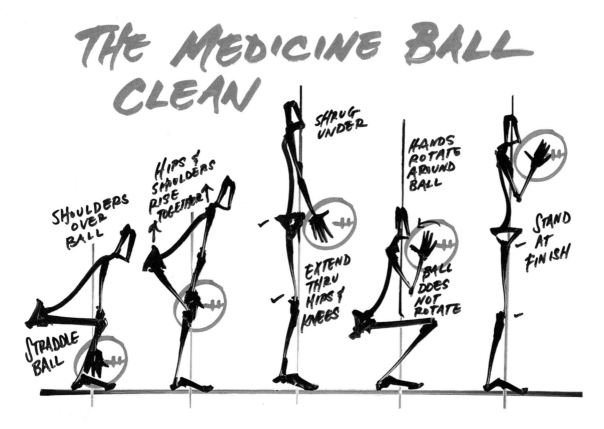

## Points of Performance

### Setup:

- Shoulder-width stance and knees in line with toes
- Ball between feet with palms on the ball
- Shoulders start over the ball

### Movement:

- Keep your trunk and neck in a neutral position.
- Keep your arms straight until your hips and legs extend.
- Bring up your hips and shoulders at the same rate; then extend your hips rapidly.
- Shrug your shoulders when you extend your hips; then pull under the medicine ball.
- Rotate your hands around the medicine ball.
- Receive the medicine ball in the bottom of a squat.
- Complete at full hip and knee extension with the ball in the front-rack position.

# THRUSTER

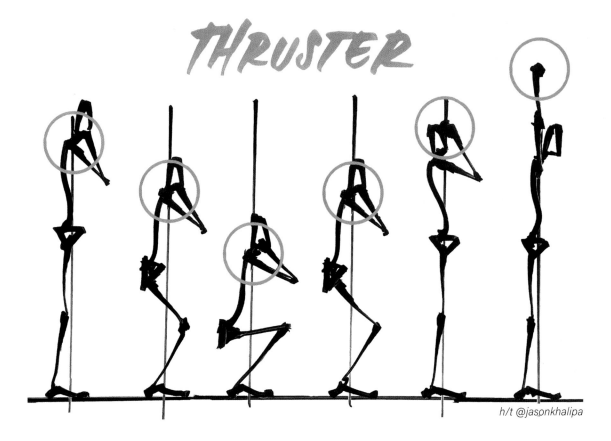

*h/t @jasonkhalipa*

## Points of Performance

### Setup:

- Shoulder-width stance
- Your hands outside of shoulder width with full grip on the bar
- The bar in the front-rack position with your elbows in front of the bar

### Movement:

- Squat by descending your hips back and down.
- Maintain a lumbar curve.
- Make sure your hips descend lower than your knees.
- Extend your hips and legs rapidly and then press.

# CHAPTER ② 

# ADAPTIVE

In this book, I'm very excited to include coaching content targeted toward the adaptive athlete, a growing demographic that deserves recognition and more attention from coaches. All the adaptive content in this book comes from the Adaptive Training Academy (ATA), a fantastic resource that was founded by a service-disabled veteran and is led by a coalition of adaptive athletes, trainers, and physios dedicated to providing research-based fitness training education.

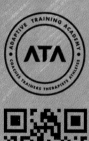

# "BOX U-TURN"
## WHEELCHAIR BOX JUMP

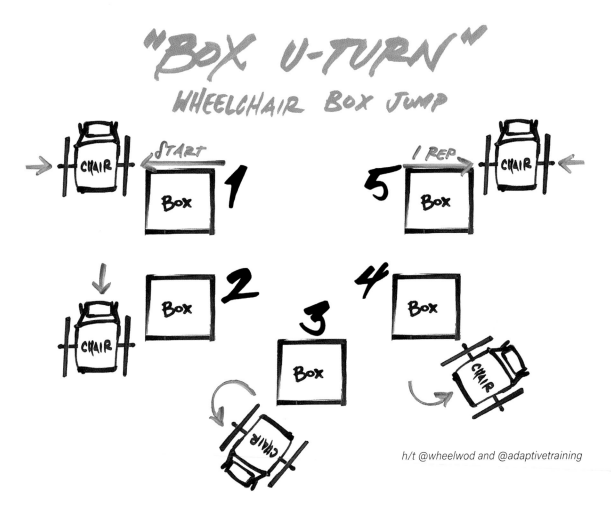

h/t @wheelwod and @adaptivetraining

## Points of Performance

### Setup:

- Start perpendicular to the edge of a box (a cone or line on the ground may also be used).
- The axle starts past the edge of a box.

### Movement:

- From the starting position, pull back.
- Spin away from the box.
- Push around the corner of the box.
- Make sure the axle clears the edge on the other side of the box.

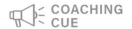
# 45° STANCE

## —WALL BALL SET UP—
## FOR UPPER EXTEMITY ATHLETE

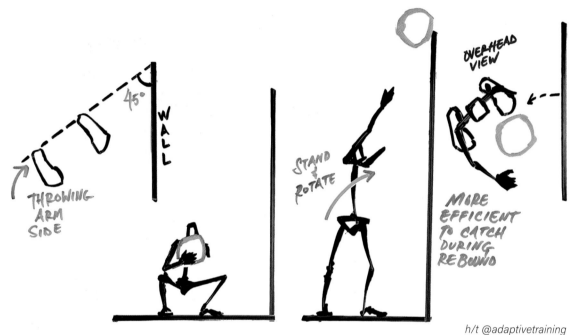

45°

WALL

THROWING ARM SIDE

STAND & ROTATE

OVERHEAD VIEW

MORE EFFICIENT TO CATCH DURING REBOUND

h/t @adaptivetraining

## When?

Wall ball shots for an upper extremity athlete

## What does this mean?

When setting up for wall ball shots, face the wall and stand an arm's distance away. Turn your stance 45° with your throwing-arm side away from the wall and the impaired side closest to the wall.

## Why is this important?

This stance provides several benefits. First, you can use rotational/transverse power to assist the throw. Second, this angle, with your impaired side closest to the target, enables you to receive the ball from the wall more efficiently. Lastly, both benefits give you more accuracy during the movement.

# SEATED ROWER
## SETUP
### — ROWING FOR ATHLETES W/O HIP MOTOR FUNCTION —

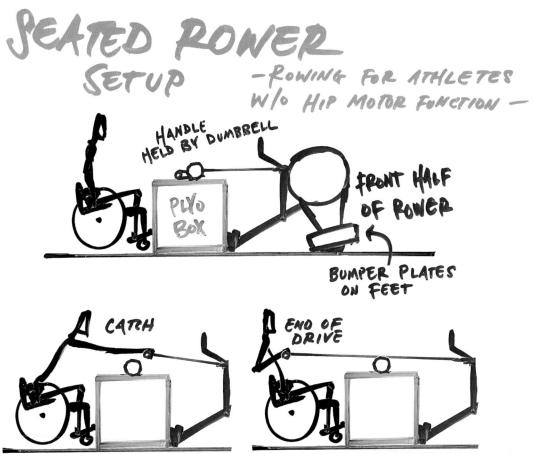

HANDLE HELD BY DUMBBELL

PLYO BOX

FRONT HALF OF ROWER

BUMPER PLATES ON FEET

CATCH

END OF DRIVE

*h/t @adaptivetraining*

## When?

Rowing for an athlete without hip motor function

## Setup:

1. Detach the monorail from the front half of the rower.
2. Place a plyo box at the base of the front half of the rower by the foot stretchers.
3. Secure the feet of the rower with weights.
4. Secure the rowing handle on the top of the box with a dumbbell.

The athlete may use the box to push against when rowing.

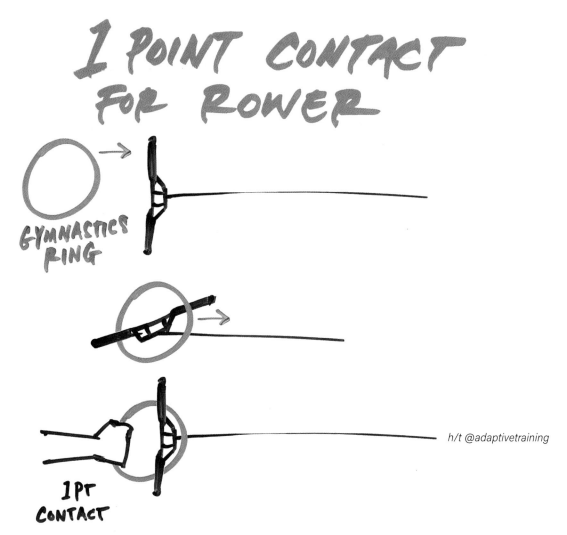

# 1 POINT CONTACT FOR ROWER

GYMNASTICS RING

1PT CONTACT

*h/t @adaptivetraining*

## When?

Rowing for an athlete with the use of only one hand

## Setup:

Pull the handle of the rower through a gymnastics ring so the tension keeps it stuck within the ring. This simple hack turns the two-handed handle into a one-contact-point option.

# "FUEL GAUGE MENTALITY"

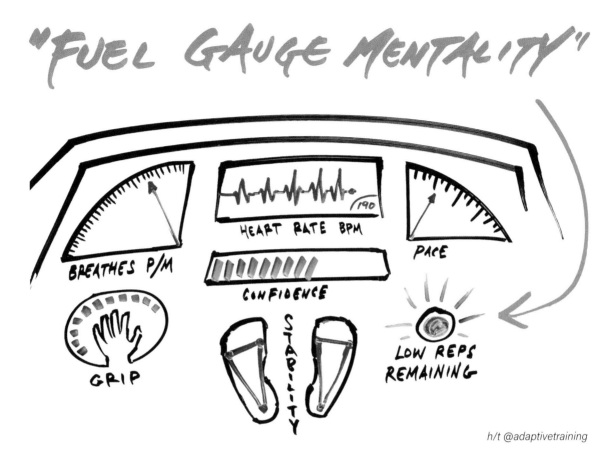

*h/t @adaptivetraining*

## What does this mean?

Cars have a light that comes on when you're supposed to stop and get more gas. It means you're running out of fuel. Your car is about to stop working.

You have a similar sensor inside your brain. You know when you only have two, three, or four reps left of a movement.

Able-bodied or standing athletes can push their bodies a little farther because they have back-up systems to catch them so they don't fall. For adaptive athletes, going to that redline has the potential to be much more dangerous.

Create an environment in your gym that promotes stopping before someone puts themselves at risk or when that gas light comes on. This is extremely important if you're working with adaptive athletes.

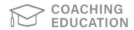
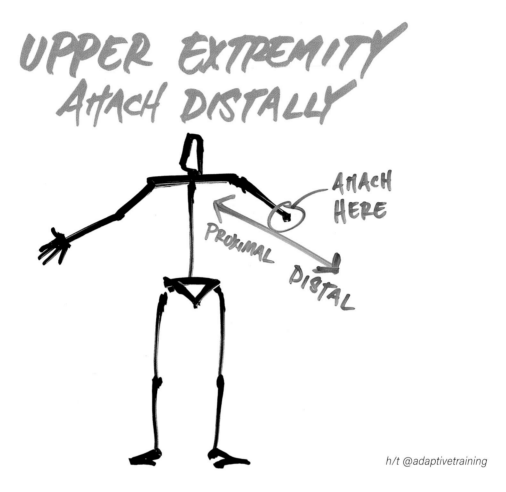

*h/t @adaptivetraining*

## When?

Upper extremity attachment

## What does this mean?

For example, don't attach at the shoulder if you can attach at the elbow. This allows the athlete to train and utilize as much of their native anatomy as possible.

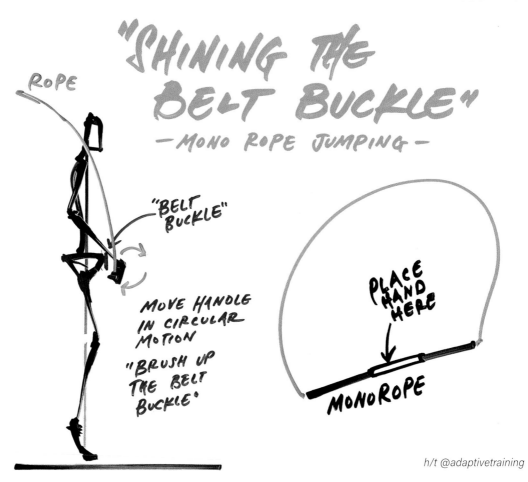

h/t @adaptivetraining

### When?

Mono rope jumping technique

### What does this mean?

When jumping rope with the mono rope, keep your hand—your one point of contact—in the middle of the handle and near your belt buckle (the center of your waist). As you jump, move your hand in a circular motion from front to back, as if you're brushing up on your belt buckle.

### Why is this important?

This motion is what keeps the momentum of the rope going to keep it traveling around your body.

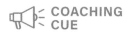
# "DRIFT OUT, DRIFT BACK"

## — GETTING MONO ROPE STARTED —

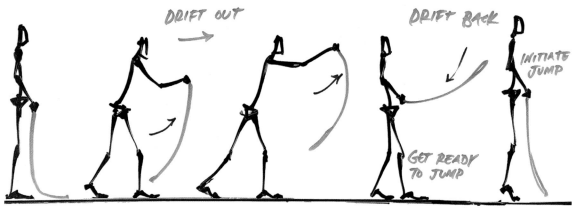

DRIFT OUT

DRIFT BACK

INITIATE
JUMP

GET READY
TO JUMP

*h/t @adaptivetraining*

## When?

Starting mono rope jump

## What does this mean?

To get started with the mono rope, take a step forward to let the rope drift away from your body and then step back to let the rope drift back toward your body. As it drifts back close to your feet, jump and carry the momentum of the rope into the first spin of the rope.

## Why is this important?

This technique allows you to get the rope moving quickly so you can start jumping.

# SEATED SNATCH
## — LAP TO OH FOR SEATED ATHLETES —

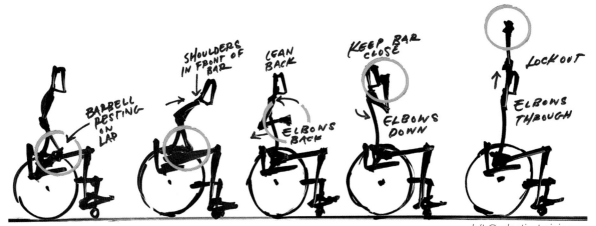

SHOULDERS IN FRONT OF BAR

BARBELL RESTING ON LAP

LEAN BACK

ELBOWS BACK

KEEP BAR CLOSE

ELBOWS DOWN

LOCKOUT

ELBOWS THROUGH

h/t @adaptivetraining

## Points of Performance

### Setup:

- Seated
- Barbell resting on lap, close to your hip crease
- Wide grip on the bar
- Arms slightly bent

### Movement:

- Lean your shoulders in front of the bar.
- Keep your arms and torso rigid and lean back.
- Drive your elbows back as the bar rises.
- As the bar rises up, drive your elbows down, through, and up.
- Press the barbell into full extension of your arms with the bar directly above your shoulders.

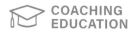
# SPOTTING A WHEELCHAIR USER

**\*ALERT**

**\* COMMUNICATION**

**\* SAFE DISTANCE**

**\* WIDE BASE OF SUPPORT**

**\* UNDERSTAND TIPPING TENDENCIES**

*h/t @adaptivetraining*

## Key Points

- **COMMUNICATION**
  - Never touch an athlete without asking permission or notifying them.
  - If you've already established the trainer/coach relationship with the athlete, you can use a simple signal, like a shoulder tap.

- **SAFETY FOR ALL**
  - The spotter needs to be in a position out of the way of the movement and out of the way if the athlete needs to bail the equipment.
  - The spotter needs to establish a wide base, with their hands on the wheelchair but away from any moving parts. The bar on the back of the wheelchair is likely a good place for the hands.

- **BE REACTIVE**
  - The spotter should not put force into the chair until they feel the chair move.

- **UNDERSTAND THE TIPPING TENDENCIES**
  - Wheelchairs are designed to be able to "pop a wheelie" to get over uneven surfaces. This also means they have the propensity to flip backward far more easily than they flip forward.
  - As the external load is lifted higher, the center of gravity rises and increases the risk of the chair and athlete flipping backward.

# APPROACHING INDIVIDUAL PROGRAMMING

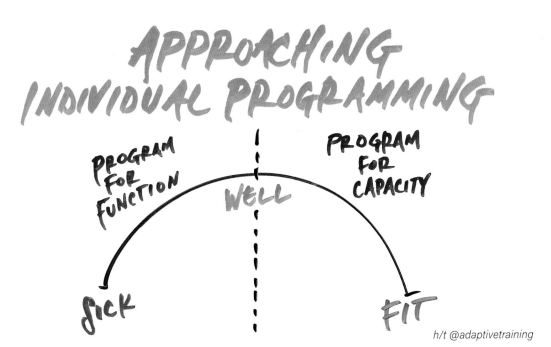

PROGRAM FOR FUNCTION

PROGRAM FOR CAPACITY

WELL

SICK

FIT

*h/t @adaptivetraining*

When programming for an individual, consider the Sickness-Wellness-Fitness continuum found in the CrossFit Level 1 Training Guide. These terms can be defined by the measurement of health indicators, such as blood pressure, body fat, cholesterol, etc. The focus of the program design is largely dependent on the current health of the athlete or where the individual is situated on the continuum.

If the individual is located on the left side of the continuum, between sickness and wellness, the focus of the program should be on functional training—in other words, training that is deliberately focused on improving the individual's quality of life. For example:

- Carrying groceries
- Avoiding falling and getting up off the ground
- Playing with their kids or grandkids
- Doing their favorite physical activity

As the individual progresses to the right, past wellness, the focus can begin to shift toward building capacity within their fitness. From a programming standpoint, this is accomplished by increasing the intensity, duration, and frequency of the training. Doing so introduces a new world of possibilities, including

- Developing capacity across training modalities
- Expanding and deepening the individual's physical skill set
- Exploring competition

# CHAPTER ③

# BRACING

# "BE PROUD TO LIFT WEIGHTS."

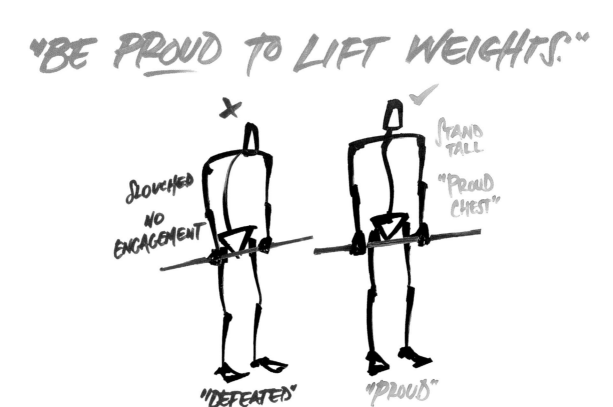

## When?

Standing while holding a barbell at the waist—deadlift lock-out, high hang clean/snatch, etc.

## What does this mean?

A common issue I see when working with novice lifters is slouched shoulders and no engagement with the upper body while holding a barbell at their waist. I tell them "Be PROUD to lift weights," which means to stand tall and have a "proud chest." Doing so engages the musculature in the upper body and helps brace the core.

## Why is this important?

Lifting weights is just as cognitive as it is physical. You must be aggressive and confident to move weight well— especially heavy weight. Standing with a "proud stance" sets you in the right position and puts you in the proper mindset.

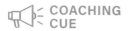

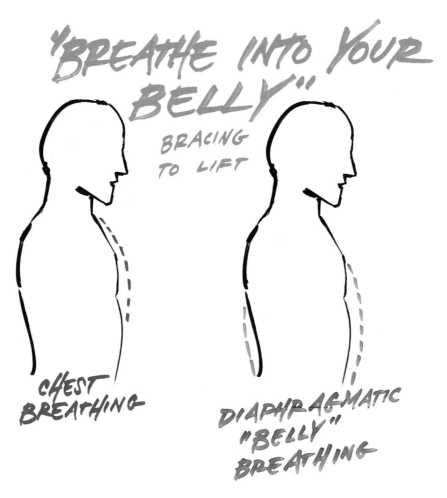

"BREATHE INTO YOUR BELLY"

BRACING TO LIFT

CHEST BREATHING

DIAPHRAGMATIC "BELLY" BREATHING

## When?

Bracing to lift

## What does this mean?

Prior to lifting anything, especially something heavy, slowly and deeply inhale as if you're filling your abdominal area. You should feel your belly expand on all sides.

## Why is this important?

Diaphragmatic breathing helps activate your core muscles and increases intra-abdominal pressure, allowing you to create and maintain a strong and stable core.

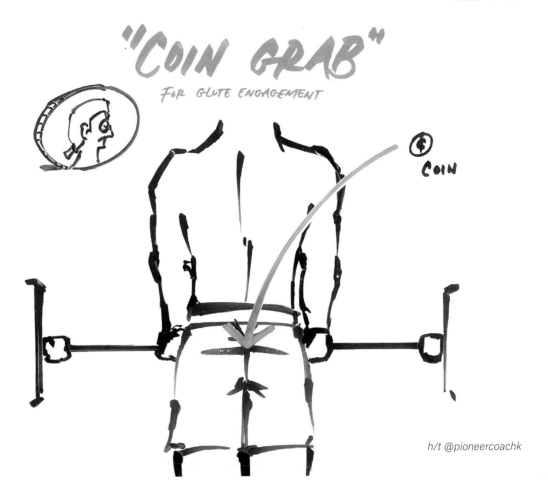

"COIN GRAB"
FOR GLUTE ENGAGEMENT

COIN

h/t @pioneercoachk

## When?

Engaging your glutes during hip extension—deadlift lock-out, the top of a kettlebell swing, glute bridges, etc.

## What does this mean?

Squeeze your glutes as if you have a coin between your butt cheeks and you want to keep it from dropping to the floor.

## Why is this important?

The glutes are the main drivers for hip extension movements and keeping you upright.

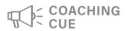
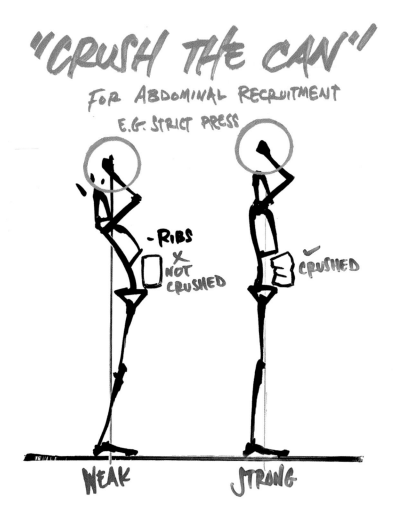

## When?

Abdominal recruitment for movements where hyperextension of the thoracic spine is a common error, including the hollow body position and pressing overhead.

## What does this mean?

Imagine a can between your hips and rib cage. You need to "crush the can."

## Why is this important?

Engaging the abdominals turns on the trifecta of "guts, butts, and quads" creating a strong column of support.

# "EXPAND YOUR SIDES"
## — BRACING TO LIFT —

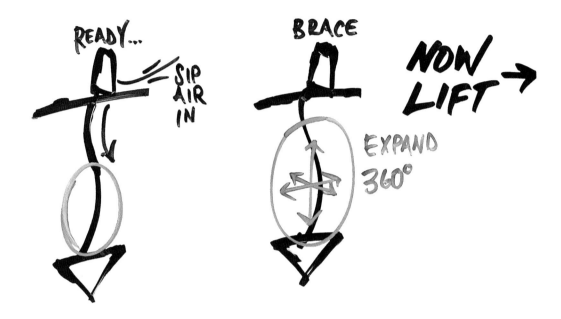

READY... SIP AIR IN

BRACE

EXPAND 360°

NOW LIFT →

## When?

Bracing to lift

## What does this mean?

Use the combination of a deep belly breath and the engagement of your core muscles to increase your intra-abdominal pressure.

You will know if you are doing this correctly by placing your hands on either side of your trunk, below your ribs and above your hip bones. As you inhale, you should feel your sides expanding and pushing your hands laterally away from your body.

## Why is this important?

When you brace, you create a strong, rigid torso, which keeps you from folding under the weight of whatever you lift or carry.

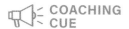
# "HOLD IN A COUGH"
## — BRACING TO LIFT —

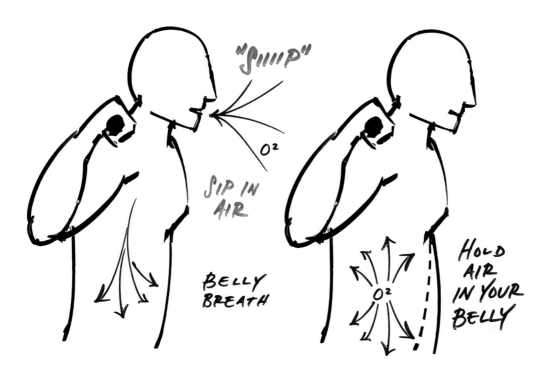

"SIIIP"

O²

SIP IN AIR

BELLY BREATH

O²

HOLD AIR IN YOUR BELLY

## When?
Bracing to lift

## What does this mean?
Before moving a barbell, take a small belly breath and pressurize your trunk by holding it in, similar to the way you would hold in a cough.

## Why is this important?
Holding in a cough creates the same type of intra-abdominal pressure needed to brace when lifting a heavy load.

# "INHALE WITHOUT RAISING THE BAR"

## BRACING TO SQUAT

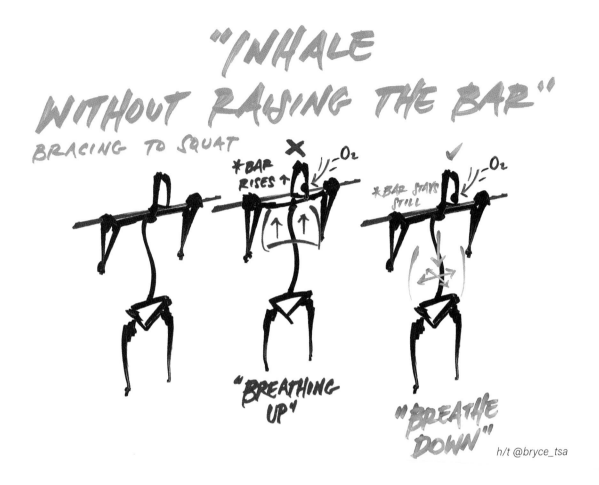

*h/t @bryce_tsa*

## When?

Bracing to squat

## What does this mean?

"Breathing up" = chest breathing = bar rises

"Breathing down" = belly breathing = bar remains still

## Why is this important?

Maximizing efficiency of a lift means minimizing any unnecessary effort. Breathing into the diaphragm fills out your belt and creates a strong, rigid core. This leads to a more efficient power transfer from the lower body into the bar.

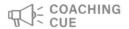
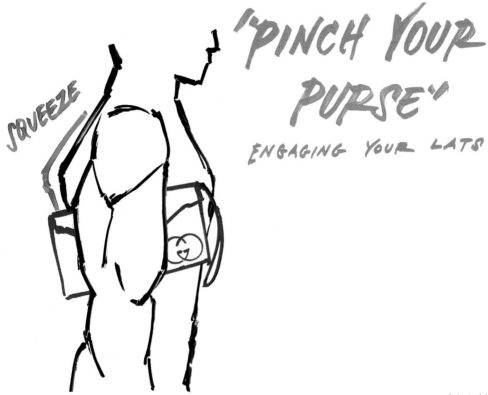

"PINCH YOUR
PURSE"
ENGAGING YOUR LATS

SQUEEZE

*h/t @thisamaesinglife_*

## When?

Engaging the lats when the elbow is inferior to the shoulder such as in athletic positions, including

- Deadlifts
- Kettlebell cleans
- Ring support position
- Jumping rope

## What does this mean?

Imagine you have a clutch purse under your armpit and you want to keep it safe.

## Why is this important?

Active shoulders are supported shoulders. Activating the lats to support your shoulders puts you in a stronger position. A common miscue is "shoulders back," which does not target engaging the strong lats and can lead to hyperextension of the torso.

# "PROTECT YOUR ARMPITS"
## - ENGAGING YOUR LATS -
### (LATISSIMUS DORSI)

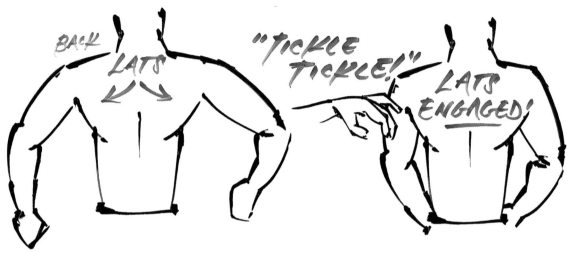

BACK
LATS
"TICKLE TICKLE!"
LATS ENGAGED!

## When?

Engaging the lats when the elbow is inferior to the shoulder as in athletic positions, including

- Deadlifts
- Kettlebell cleans
- Ring support position
- Jumping rope
- Engaging the lats during bench press

## What does this mean?

Imagine someone is trying to tickle your armpit, and you are squeezing your armpit shut. A common miscue is "shoulders back," which does not target engaging the strong lats and can lead to hyperextension of the torso.

## Why is this important?

By doing this motion, you engage your latissimus dorsi and create an active shoulder. Active shoulders are supported shoulders. Activating the lats to support your shoulders puts you in a stronger position.

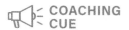
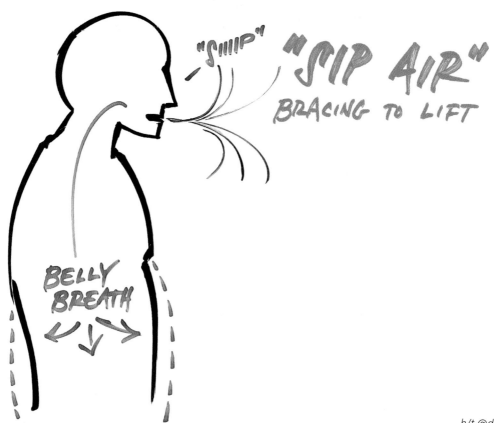

*h/t @dozer.wl*

## When?
Bracing to lift

## What does this mean?
When you brace for a lift, taking a wide-open gulp of air can result in breathing into your ribs. Doing so does not provide proper bracing for lifting heavy weight.

Instead, forcefully sipping air properly increases your intra-abdominal pressure and prepares your torso to lift heavy weight.

## Why is this important?
Bracing for a lift involves properly increasing the intra-abdominal pressure of your core.

# "TURN ON THE BBQ"

### ENGAGE BELLY, BUTT, & QUADS
### E.G. PUSH PRESS SETUP

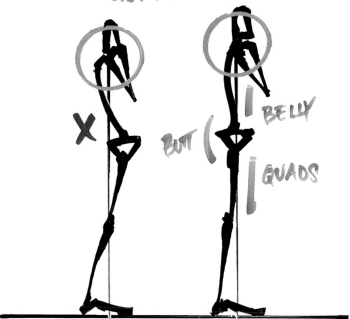

*h/t @coachjasonackerman*

## When?

Engaging the core

## What does this mean?

Create a strong column of support by turning on the BBQ: engage your belly, butt, and quads. For example,

- Setting up for a push press, turn on the BBQ.

- Lock out a deadlift, turn on the BBQ.

- Pressing out a handstand, turn on the BBQ.

# CHAPTER ④

## DEADLIFT

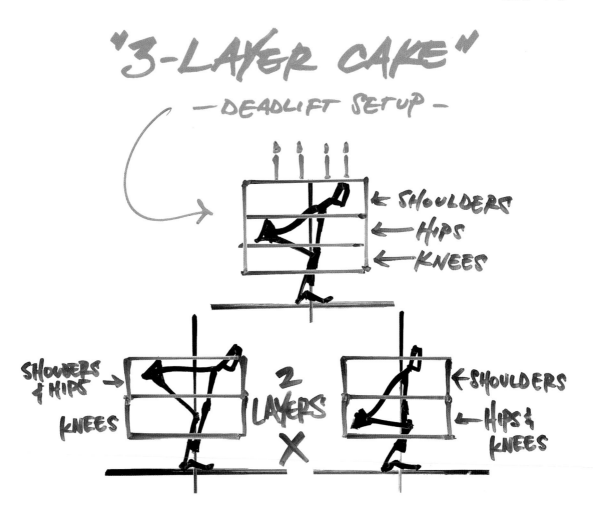

# "3-LAYER CAKE"
## — DEADLIFT SETUP —

SHOULDERS
HIPS
KNEES

SHOULDERS & HIPS
KNEES

2 LAYERS
X

SHOULDERS
HIPS & KNEES

## When?

Setup for a deadlift

## What does this mean?

During the setup for the deadlift, the knees, hips, and shoulders should each be in their own layer. Of course, the angle of the back varies slightly based on the athlete's limb length. However, the hips should be higher than the knees, and the shoulders should be higher than the hips.

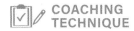

# THE DEADLIFT IN 5 STEPS

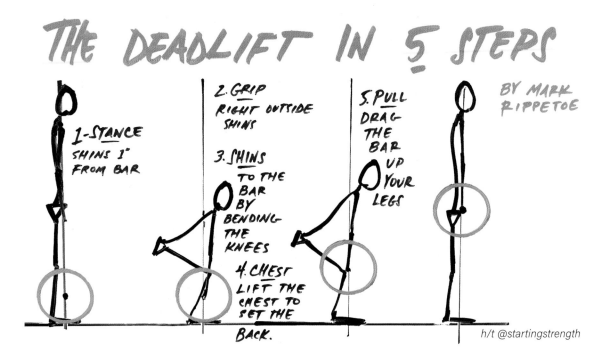

1 - STANCE SHINS 1" FROM BAR

2. GRIP RIGHT OUTSIDE SHINS

3. SHINS TO THE BAR BY BENDING THE KNEES

4. CHEST LIFT THE CHEST TO SET THE BACK.

5. PULL DRAG THE BAR UP YOUR LEGS

BY MARK RIPPETOE

h/t @startingstrength

## When?

Deadlifting

## What does this mean?

1. **Feet:** Step up to the bar so your mid-foot is directly under the bar and your stance is hip width. DO NOT MOVE THE BARBELL because doing so changes the spatial relationship of your body and the bar, negating the purpose of the setup.

2. **Hands:** Bend at your hips and place your hands on the bar with a shoulder-width grip. Your arms should be parallel, and your hands should be directly below your shoulders. DO NOT MOVE THE BARBELL.

3. **Shins:** Bend your knees so your shins are gently touching the barbell. This places your hips in the correct position. DO NOT MOVE THE BARBELL.

4. **Chest:** Squeeze your chest out. Doing so engages the muscles in your torso, especially your powerful lats. It also sets tension in your body, priming your central nervous system to lift. DO NOT MOVE THE BARBELL.

5. **Push:** Squeeze the bar and push your feet into the ground. Keep the bar as close to your body as you can.

## Why is this important?

Just like with any lift, a better start leads to a better finish.

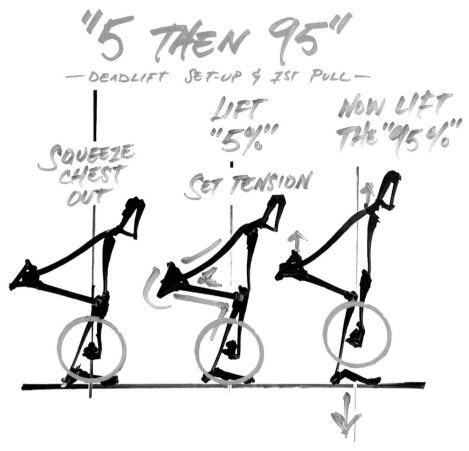

# "5 THEN 95"
## — DEADLIFT SET-UP & 1ST PULL —

SQUEEZE CHEST OUT

LIFT "5%"

SET TENSION

NOW LIFT THE "95%"

## When?

Deadlift setup and first pull

## What does this mean?

During the deadlift setup, prior to the liftoff, pull up on the bar as if you are lifting 5 percent of the weight. By doing so, you will set tension through your body and take out the slack of the bar.

Once you have done this, NOW lift the remaining 95 percent.

## Why is this important?

The deadlift doesn't start with an eccentric lowering of the weight, which makes it more difficult to brace prior to lifting. Taking a moment to brace properly prior to lifting the weight off the ground can make a huge difference.

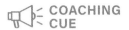 

# "CLICK, THEN COLLECT"

## DURING DEADLIFT

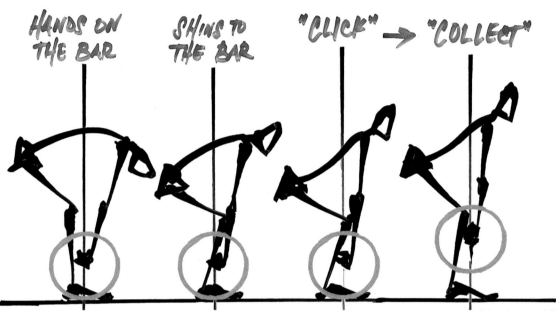

HANDS ON THE BAR     SHINS TO THE BAR     "CLICK" → "COLLECT"

h/t @jeanpauldk

## When?

Deadlift

## What does this mean?

Click the bar and THEN collect the weights to create tension before you lift the weight off the ground.

During the setup, squeeze the bar, engage your lats, and feel even and full foot pressure. Doing so will make the bar click. THEN push your feet into the ground to lift the bar.

## Why is this important?

The deadlift doesn't start with an eccentric lowering of the weight, which makes it more difficult to brace prior to lifting. Taking a moment to brace properly prior to lifting the weight off the ground will make a huge difference.

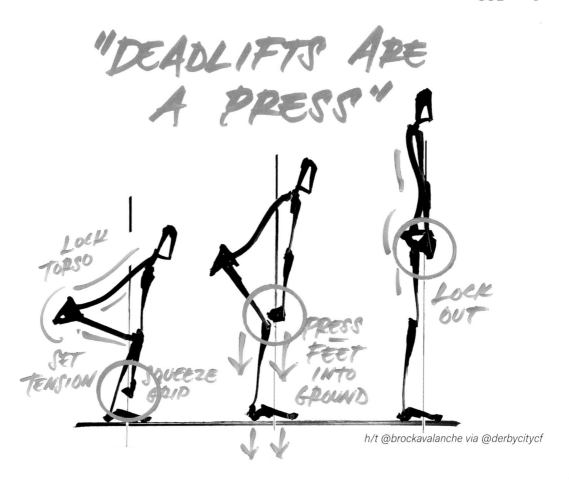

# "DEADLIFTS ARE A PRESS"

LOCK TORSO

SET TENSION

SQUEEZE GRIP

PRESS = FEET INTO GROUND

LOCK OUT

*h/t @brockavalanche via @derbycitycf*

## What does this mean?

Quite often, people think of the deadlift as pulling the bar off the ground. Doing so places a focus on using your back.

Instead, think of the deadlift as holding on to the bar and pressing your feet into the ground as if you are squatting the earth away.

## Why is this important?

Visualizing the deadlift as a press with the legs engages the strong musculature of your lower body to work together with your back and core to lift the weight.

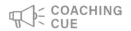
# "DON'T BREAK THE EGGS"

## — TOUCH & GO DEADLIFTS —

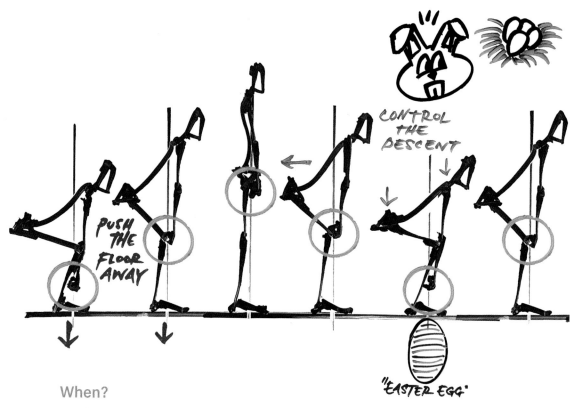

PUSH THE FLOOR AWAY

CONTROL THE DESCENT

"EASTER EGG"

## When?

Touch-and-go deadlifts

## What does this mean?

There are two sides to the movement of a muscle contraction. Lifting weight, when the muscles shorten, is the concentric muscle contraction. Lowering weight, when the muscle lengthens, is the eccentric muscle contraction.

Think about tapping the weights on the floor like you are touching an egg shell. Don't break it!

## Why is this important?

During the deadlift, lifting the bar is only half of the rep. Lowering the bar with control provides massive benefit to building strength. Maintain complete control throughout the entire rep.

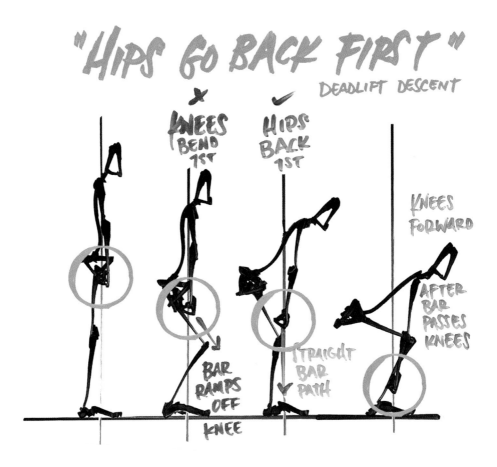

# "HIPS GO BACK FIRST"
### DEADLIFT DESCENT

✗ KNEES BEND 1ST

✓ HIPS BACK 1ST

KNEES FORWARD

AFTER BAR PASSES KNEES

BAR RAMPS OFF KNEE

STRAIGHT BAR PATH

## When?
Deadlift descent

## What does this mean?
Just as the bar path during the lift of the deadlift should be straight, the bar path during the descent should be straight.

From the top, locked out position, allow the hips to go back first, into a hinge position.

## Why is this important?
This movement provides a straight bar path for the bar to return to the ground. Your knees travel forward once the bar passes them.

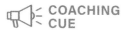
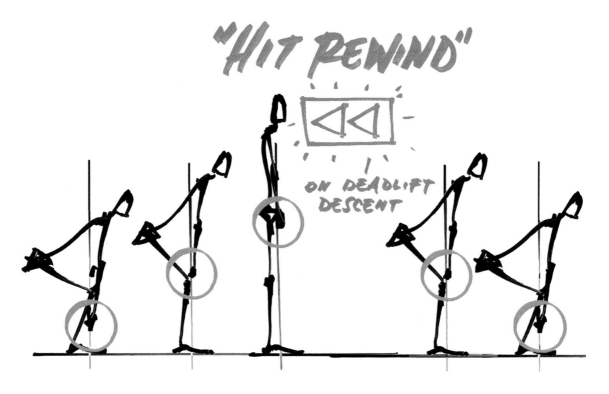

## When?

Lowering the bar during the deadlift

## What does this mean?

A common error among novice weightlifters when lowering the bar during the deadlift is initiating the movement with a squat pattern. By doing so, the bar path inefficiently travels forward and around the knee.

To fix this, the lifter needs to follow the same movement pattern but in reverse (hinge and then lower the bar). Once the lifter demonstrates proper mechanics when lifting the bar to lockout, cue them to "hit rewind" to lower the bar.

## Why is this important?

Understanding that the movement pattern of the deadlift is the same on the concentric (lifting) as it is on the eccentric (lowering) simplifies the movement and helps the lifter move more efficiently.

# "KNEES INTO ELBOWS"
## — DEADLIFT SETUP —

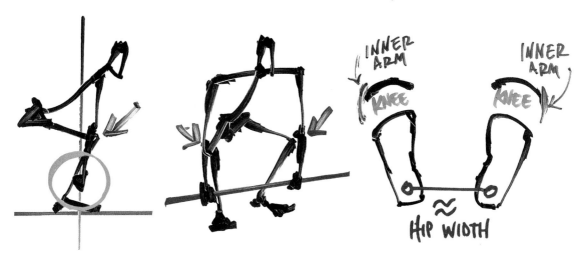

INNER ARM
KNEE

INNER ARM
KNEE

≈ HIP WIDTH

## When?

Start position for deadlift

## What does this mean?

During the deadlift setup, your feet should be in a hip-width stance with your toes pointing slightly outward (think 11:00 and 1:00). Hand placement on the bar should be so your arms hang vertically. Bend your knees forward until your shins touch the bar. Push your chest out and press your knees into your elbows.

## Why is this important?

Pressing your knees into your elbows does the following:

- Keeps your knees in line with your toes
- Moves your thighs out of the way for your belly
- Externally rotates your hips to recruit more adductor into the movement
- Sets your hips in an optimal position for back extension
- Helps create tension through your body and take the slack out of the bar

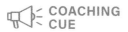
# "MAKE THE BAR HOVER"
## DEADLIFT SET UP

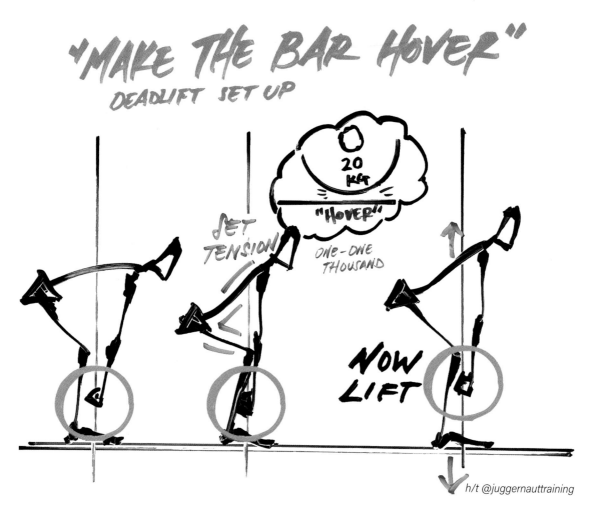

SET TENSION

20 KG

"HOVER"

ONE - ONE THOUSAND

NOW LIFT

*h/t @juggernauttraining*

## When?
Deadlift setup

## What does this mean?
Prior to initiating the lift, squeeze into position by barely pulling up on the bar, as if you are making the bar hover.

## Why is this important?
Doing so allows you to set tension throughout your body, similar to the feeling of holding the weight at the top of a squat. Setting tension connects your body to the bar and prepares your body to brace and lift.

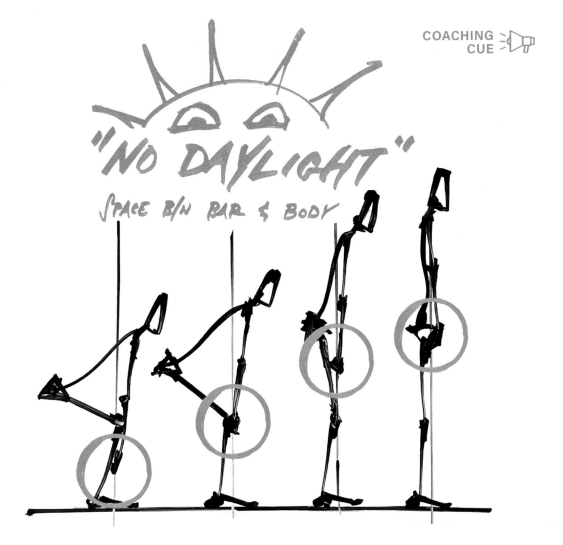

"NO DAYLIGHT"
SPACE B/N BAR & BODY

## When?

Barbell deadlifts

## What does this mean?

How close should you keep the barbell during deadlifts? There should be "no daylight" between the barbell and your body. Keep the barbell as close to the body as possible without cutting your shins.

## Why is this important?

The farther the weight is from the midline, the harder you will work to control the weight. To keep the bar path efficient, keep it as close as possible.

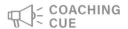
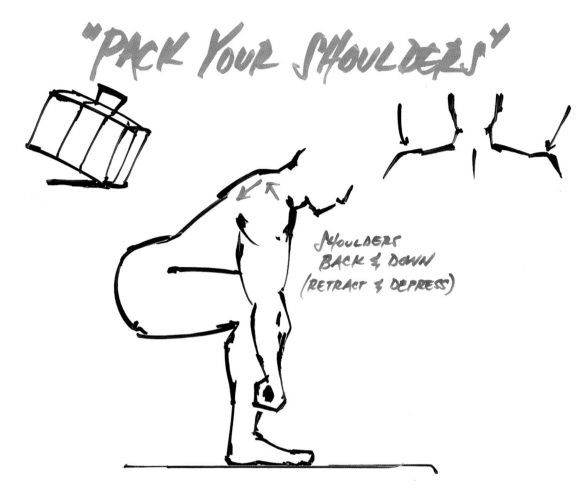

"PACK YOUR SHOULDERS"

SHOULDERS
BACK & DOWN
(RETRACT & DEPRESS)

## When?

During the setup for deadlifts, cleans, etc.

## What does this mean?

To "pack your shoulders" draw them back and down (retract and depress them) away from your ears. You will feel them packed solid and tight against your torso. This will engage your lats and prepare your upper back to lift heavy weight.

## Why is this important?

A strong setup position must engage the muscles in the upper back before the lifter moves the bar off the ground.

# "PULL YOUR HIPS DOWN"
## —DEADLIFT SETUP—

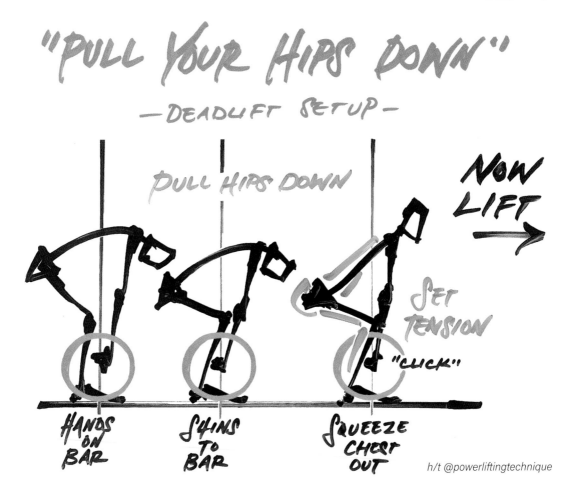

PULL HIPS DOWN

NOW LIFT →

SET TENSION

"CLICK"

HANDS ON BAR

SHINS TO BAR

SQUEEZE CHEST OUT

*h/t @powerliftingtechnique*

## When?

Deadlift setup

## What does this mean?

After gripping the bar, as you bring your hips down to the barbell, think about squeezing your glutes and hamstrings as hard as possible.

## Why is this important?

The deadlift doesn't have an eccentric range of motion when starting. You're pulling from a dead stop, and your muscles don't get the opportunity to create tension. Therefore, you must actively create lower body tension in your deadlift setup. Without it, you'll struggle to get the weight off the floor.

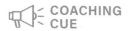
# "PULL WITH THE LEGS"
## — PICKING WEIGHT UP OFF THE GROUND —

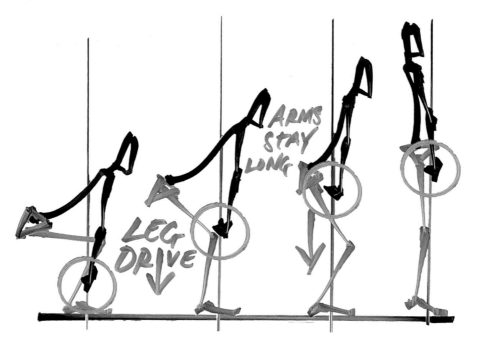

ARMS
STAY
LONG

LEG
DRIVE

## When?

Picking up weight from the ground (e.g., deadlift, clean, snatch, etc.)

## What does this mean?

The initial movement of the clean, snatch, and deadlift is called the first pull. Unfortunately, yet understandably, most people think of arm flexion when told to pull. However, this is the opposite of what should happen. Instead, keep arms long, torso rigid, and drive with your legs through the first pull.

## Why is this important?

Driving with the legs through the first pull keeps the power coming from the powerful lower body.

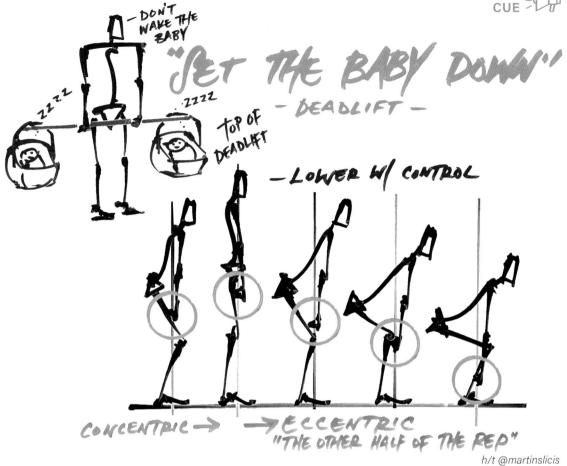

DON'T WAKE THE BABY

ZZZZ   ZZZZ

TOP OF DEADLIFT

"SET THE BABY DOWN"
— DEADLIFT —

— LOWER W/ CONTROL

CONCENTRIC → → ECCENTRIC
"THE OTHER HALF OF THE REP"

*h/t @martinslicis*

## When?

Deadlift

## What does this mean?

When training the deadlift, lower the bar with control.

Many novice lifters mistake the lockout of the deadlift for the completion of a rep and then drop the bar back to the floor.

Doing so foolishly leaves the lifter without the benefit of gains to be made by lowering the bar with control.

## Why is this important?

There are two segments to deadlift (or any lift, for that matter), both of equal importance: the lifting (concentric) and the lowering (eccentric). To maximize the benefit, focus on controlling both portions of the lift.

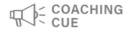

## COACHING CUE

# "TAKE THE SLACK OUT OF THE BAR."

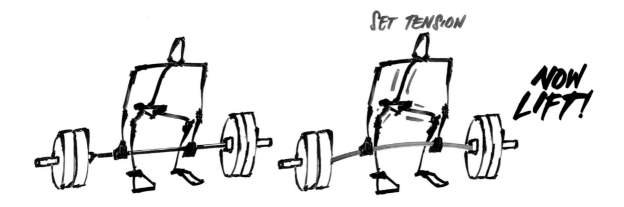

SET TENSION

NOW LIFT!

## When?

Prior to lifting off the ground (deadlift, clean, snatch, etc.)

## What does this mean?

Once your stance, grip, and position are set, create tension through your body by very slightly pulling up on the bar. By doing so, you will take the slack out of the bar (the bend that occurs during the lift), as well as create a connection from the bar THROUGH your body and INTO the floor.

## Why is this important?

This simple step helps send a message from the mind to the body that says, "We are about to lift something heavy. Get ready!"

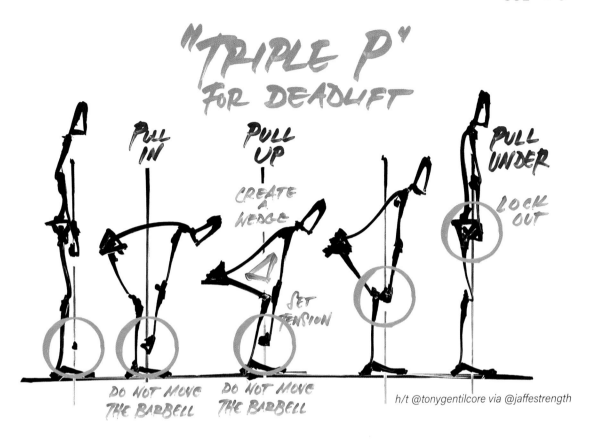

"TRIPLE P" FOR DEADLIFT

PULL IN

PULL UP
CREATE A WEDGE
SET TENSION

PULL UNDER
LOCK OUT

DO NOT MOVE THE BARBELL

DO NOT MOVE THE BARBELL

h/t @tonygentilcore via @jaffestrength

## When?

Deadlift

## What does this mean?

Take your time with your deadlift setup. Get the most out each rep by being methodical with your approach and execution by using the Triple P:

- PULL IN: Pull yourself in to the bar.

- PULL UP: Use the barbell as a counterbalance to "wedge" yourself in place and to gain more thoracic extension.

- PULL UNDER: At lockout, many lifters think "pull back" and end up hyper-extending through their low back. This results in soft knees at lockout and poor leverage. Instead, think about locking the hips UNDERNEATH the bar

I like a fourth P, between pull up and pull under: PUSH AWAY: Push your feet into the floor.

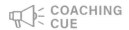

# "VERTICAL & PARALLEL ARMS"
## — DEADLIFT SETUP —

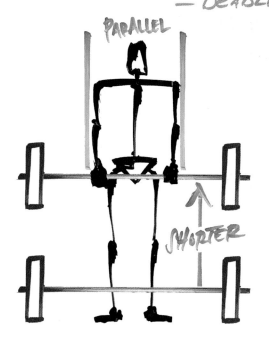

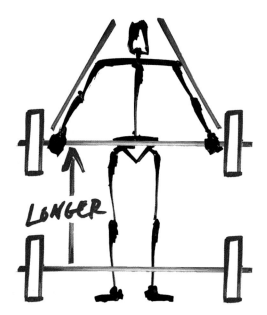

## When?

Deadlift (conventional or sumo) setup

## What does this mean?

Grip width on the barbell should allow for your arms to hang vertically and parallel to each other.

## Why is this important?

This setup enables you to efficiently complete a rep with the shortest bar path. A wider grip (that is, snatch grip) requires the bar to travel a farther distance.

# "SQUAT THEN HINGE"
## — DEADLIFT —

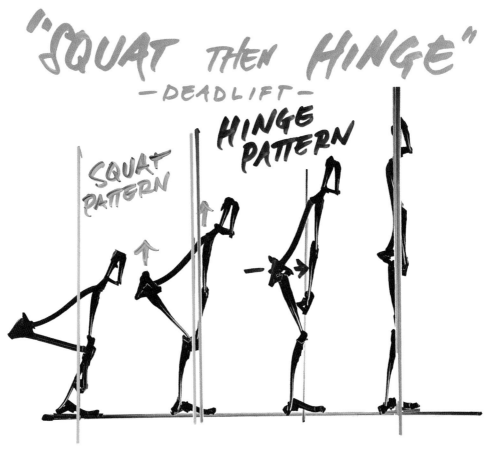

SQUAT PATTERN

HINGE PATTERN

## When?

Deadlift

## What does this mean?

The deadlift movement sequence is a squat then a hinge.

During the initial lift, the movement is a squat pattern. Your hips and shoulders rise at the same rate. Once the bar passes your knees, your hips drive forward, and your trunk moves upright.

During the descent, you reverse the movement pattern: hinge until the bar reaches your knees and then squat the bar back down to the floor.

## Why is this important?

Breaking down a movement to smaller, simpler movements can make it easier for athletes to understand how to move efficiently.

# CHAPTER ⑤

# EDUCATION

# MOVEMENT

## "ENERGY LEAK"

— MOVEMENT INEFFICIENCY —
E.G. BACK SQUAT

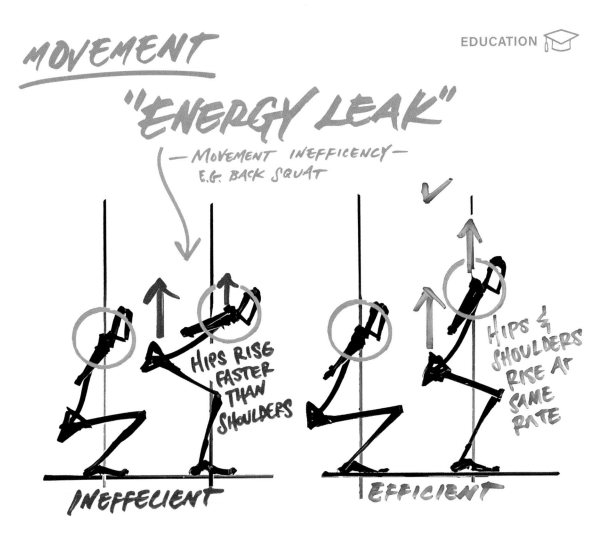

HIPS RISE FASTER THAN SHOULDERS

HIPS & SHOULDERS RISE AT SAME RATE

INEFFICIENT

EFFICIENT

## What does this mean?

An energy leak is a movement inefficiency that occurs when the thing being moved doesn't move at the same rate as the body part moving it.

For example, during the ascent of the squat, an energy leak occurs if the hips move faster than the barbell.

**The thing being moved:** The barbell/shoulders (the barbell is located at the shoulders)

**The body part moving it:** The hips

## Why is this important?

Efficient movement uses minimum effort to provide the maximum output. If a body part is moving but the weight is not, you're wasting effort. To maximize performance, you must understand the importance of moving efficiently.

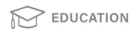
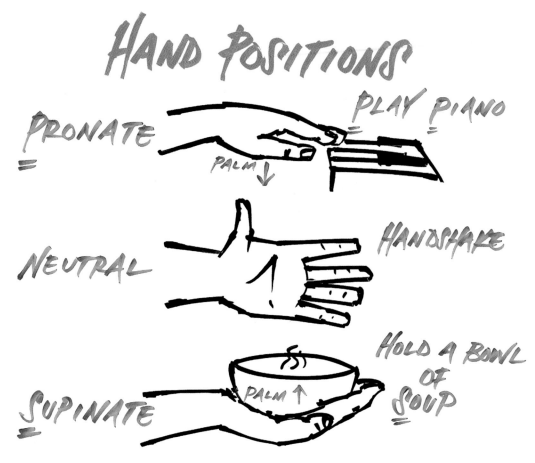

## Describing hand positions:

- **Pronation:** Play piano
- **Neutral:** Handshake
- **Supination:** Bowl of soup

## What does this mean?

The following alliteration cues can be used to remember anatomical hand positions:

- To *play piano*, you *pronate* your hands.
- To hold a bowl of **soup**, you *supinate* your hands.

# MOVEMENT CORRECTION

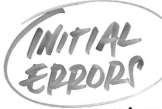

**INITIAL ERRORS** — CREATE → **SUBSEQUENT ERRORS**

FOCUS ON THESE FIRST

E.G. UNEVEN BALANCE

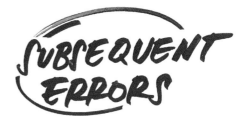

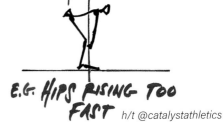

E.G. HIPS RISING TOO FAST

*h/t @catalystathletics*

## What does this mean?

When an athlete displays multiple errors during a movement, and they commonly will, it is important to focus on the errors that occur earliest in the sequence. Correcting these will likely fix errors that happen afterward. I have found this to be true regardless of the sport (Olympic weightlifting, rowing, gymnastics, etc.).

## Why is this important?

Efficiently correcting an error might require that you take a closer look at the movement pattern and identify what could be causing the issue further down the chain. The majority of the time, the initial source of the subsequent errors stems from an issue with balance through the feet. A broad order of operations that I use for tracing the source of a problem is

- Stance
- Grip
- Position

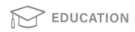 

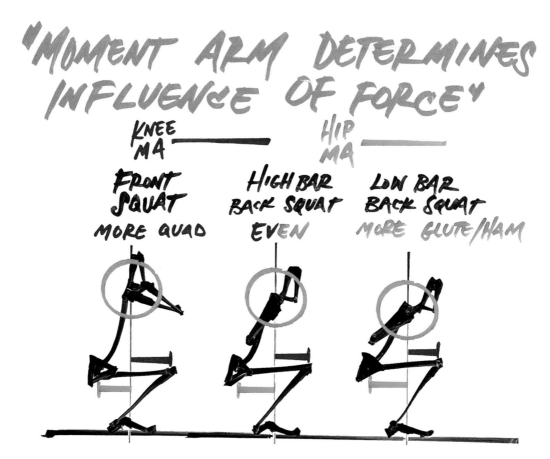

## "MOMENT ARM DETERMINES INFLUENCE OF FORCE"

KNEE MA ———

HIP MA ———

| FRONT SQUAT | HIGH BAR BACK SQUAT | LOW BAR BACK SQUAT |
| MORE QUAD | EVEN | MORE GLUTE/HAM |

## What does this mean?

A moment arm is simply the length between a joint axis and the line of force acting on that joint. In other words, how your body moves when lifting weight determines which muscles are taxed.

## Examples:

**Red line = Knee moment arm:**
Quad dominant

**Green line = Hip moment arm:**
Glute/hamstring dominant

- Front squat: Slightly more quad dominant
- High bar back squat: Relatively equal force
- Low bar back squat: Slightly more glute/hamstring dominant

## Why is this important?

*How* you lift determines how *much* you lift. You need to understand the biomechanics of your body and how it plays a role in moving efficiently.

  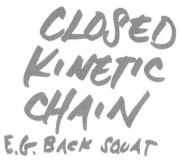

# OPEN KINETIC CHAIN
E.G. BENCH PRESS

# CLOSED KINETIC CHAIN
E.G. BACK SQUAT

VS.

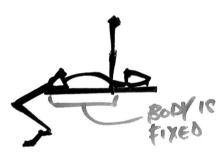
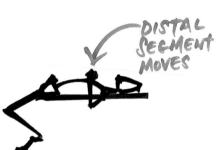
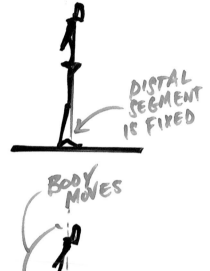

## What does this mean?

**Open kinetic chain:** The body is fixed, and the distal segment moves—for example, bench press.

**Closed kinetic chain:** The distal segment is fixed and the body moves—for example, back squat

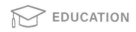 

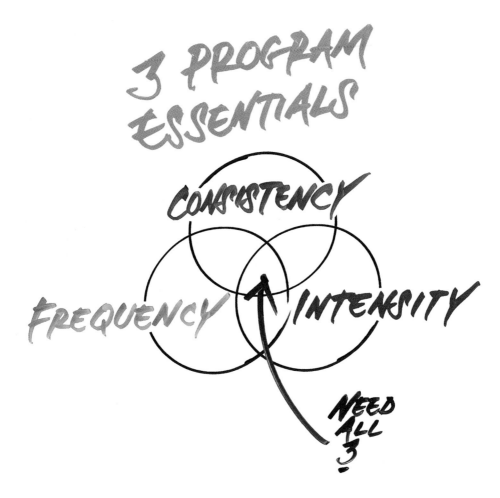

## What does this mean?

Regardless of the activity (CrossFit, Olympic weightlifting, powerlifting, Orange Theory, Zumba, etc.), you must have three elements to see progress: consistency, frequency, and intensity. Each of these elements are relative to the individual.

- **Consistency:** Keep your training a priority within your daily/weekly routine just as you make it a priority to brush your teeth daily.

- **Frequency:** Training every single Wednesday may be consistent, but it certainly isn't frequent. Three days a week is the recommended minimum for physical training.

- **Intensity:** For the body to adapt to a stimulus, there must be at least some stress. Stress and recovery are synergists and work together.

# "ANTHROPOMETRICS"
## AN-THRUH-PUH-MEH-TRIKS

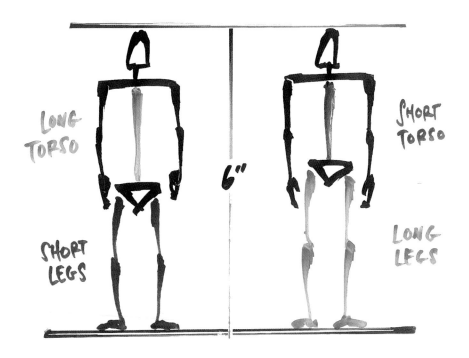

## What is this?

Anthropometrics is the science of measuring size and proportions of the human body.

It's easy to understand that each human body is built differently from the next, some more so than others. Therefore, it should also be understood that no two athletes will move EXACTLY the same way.

Since the laws of physics are consistent, each athlete must move in accordance to their own body proportions.

Coaches, keep this in mind when working with your athletes.

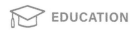 

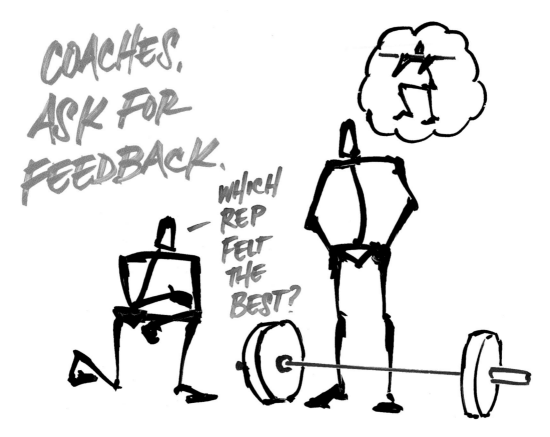

## What does this mean?

When working with my athletes, I often ask them for feedback immediately after a set/rep:

- "How did that last rep feel?"
- "Which rep felt the best? Why?"
- "Where did that bar path go? Why?"
- "Could you tell a difference?" (after I've provided a cue)

## Why is this important?

When an athlete is asked to provide verbal feedback, they're forced to pay attention to their movement, which helps them strengthen their mind and body awareness and create a deeper understanding of an efficient movement pattern (rather than just "going through the motions.")

# COACHES, YOU ARE NOT "BAD WITH NAMES."

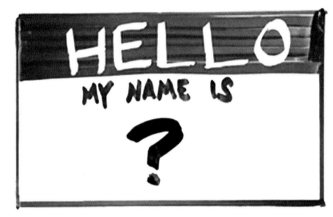

## What does this mean?

Coaches are leaders. Leaders direct and organize people.

What is worse?

Humbling yourself and asking an athlete's name that you should know

OR

Continuing to call them "bud," "dude," "mate," "champ," or "kiddo."

Try using pre-class ice breakers:

- Writing names down on a whiteboard

- Repeating someone's name three or four times out loud

## Why is this important?

One cannot effectively direct and organize others in a small group setting if they do not know/use people's names. Work on your name-memory like you would your squat.

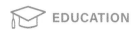
# "THE CANDLE ANALOGY"
## DESCRIBING RELATIVE TRAINING INTENSITY

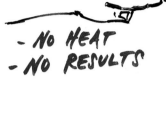

- NO HEAT
- NO RESULTS

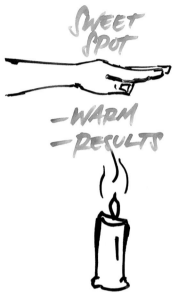

SWEET SPOT

- WARM
- RESULTS

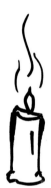

- TOO HOT
- INJURY

*h/t @apbozman via @variednotrandom*

## When?

Describing relative training intensity

## What does this mean?

Think of the proximity between your hand and a lit candle as a measure of intensity. If you hold your hand so far above the flame that you don't feel any heat, the intensity is so low you can continue doing this forever and nothing will happen. On the opposite side, if you hold your hand so close to the flame that you immediately get burned, the intensity is far too high and quickly causes injury.

The sweet spot is to find the distance between your hand and the candle where you can continuously hold it and feel the warmth. This level of intensity provides you with the most benefit. The same applies to relative intensity during training.

# COACH "HANDS FREE"

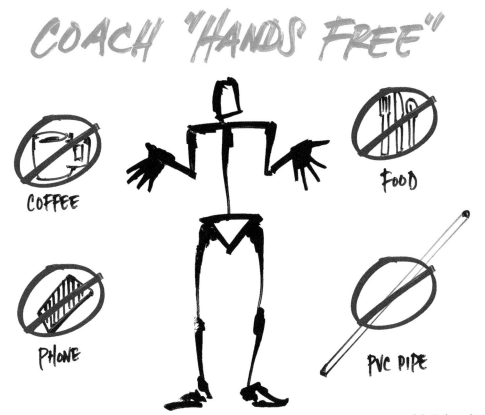

COFFEE

FOOD

PHONE

PVC PIPE

*h/t @clcoachtocoach*

## What does this mean?

Body language speaks LOUDLY, especially for those who coach movement. Your athlete(s) should be your main focus while you are coaching. Keep your hands free whenever you are coaching.

**Examples of "hands full" coaching:**

- Scrolling on your phone
- Drinking coffee
- Eating
- Hands in pockets
- Carrying around a PVC pipe (use it only when you need it)

## Why is this important?

Being distracted by your phone, a snack, or something you're fiddling with damages your relationship with your athletes.

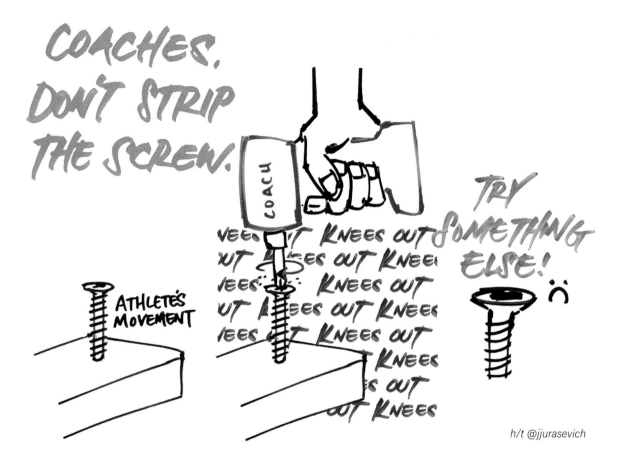

COACHES, DON'T STRIP THE SCREW.

h/t @jjurasevich

## What does this mean?

If you are using a cue with an athlete and do not see improvement, do not continue using that same cue. Try something new.

## Why is this important?

Every athlete is different, and each responds in their own way to coaching cues or a method. It is the coach's job to employ the best approach for each athlete.

# EXAMPLES OF "WHITE NOISE"

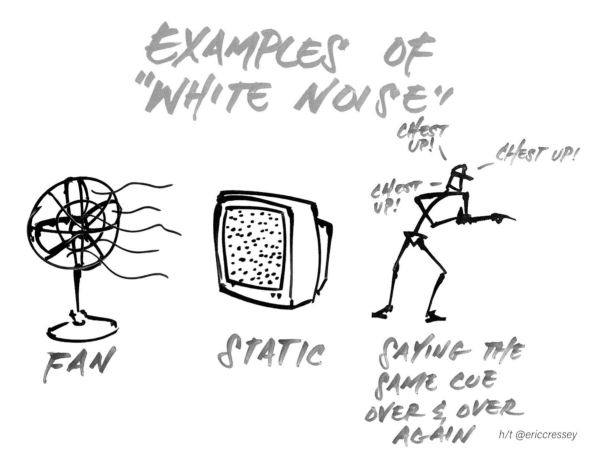

FAN

STATIC

SAYING THE SAME CUE OVER & OVER AGAIN

*h/t @ericcressey*

### When?

Providing feedback while coaching

### What does this mean?

"White noise" is background noise. It is a constant and predictable sound.

When you coach, are your cues predictable phrases that you've always used, regardless of the outcome? Do you only use cues that make sense to you? Or are you providing valuable, individualized feedback based on the performance of your athlete?

### Why is this important?

Athletes need clear, concise cues specific to their individual needs. If you can't provide this kind of cue, it's better to stay silent than give them a generic, repetitive cue. If you're saying the same cue over and over again without seeing a change in the athlete, you need to find different cue or method for explaining the desired outcome.

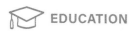
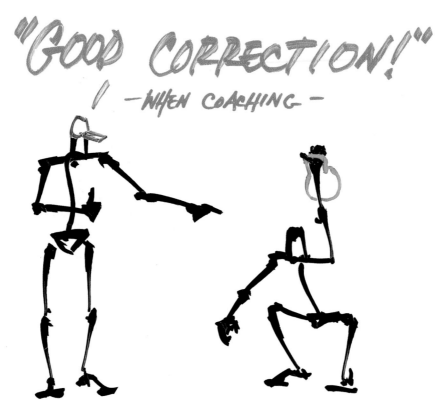

"GOOD CORRECTION!"
— WHEN COACHING —

## When?

Providing feedback while coaching

## What does this mean?

Simply put, if you see your athlete make a correction on their own, especially if it addresses a weakness of theirs, let the athlete know. For example, "Good correction! I like how you braced before you moved."

An effective coach never wastes a rep. They use every opportunity to help their athletes move better.

## Why is this important?

Often, especially when working with beginners, it can be easy for a coach to focus on faults and provide cues to improve them. When an athlete reaches the point of making the correction on their own, the coach should acknowledge this. Providing affirmation like this helps the athlete develop a stronger kinesthetic awareness and mind/body connection.

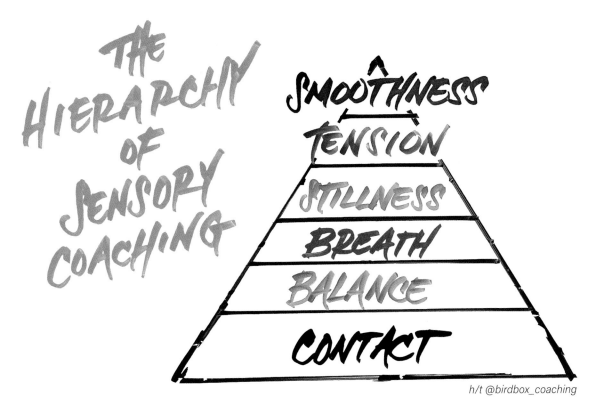

THE HIERARCHY OF SENSORY COACHING

SMOOTHNESS
TENSION
STILLNESS
BREATH
BALANCE
CONTACT

*h/t @birdbox_coaching*

## What does this mean?

The six key sensory steps toward becoming a coaching master:

1. **Contact:** The main anchor point (e.g., feet on the ground, hands on the bar, etc.). The integrity and understanding of this contact point affects the quality and efficiency of the entire movement.

2. **Balance:** The center point of the athlete. The place where the distribution of the athlete's ability and skill can be executed with maximum output and efficiency.

3. **Breath:** The breath gives structure and energy to facilitate all athletic movement. The breath prepares the athlete before and/or during each physical action.

4. **Stillness:** This is the combined result of contact, balance, and breath. The application of stillness displays control before and/or during the expression of the physical action.

5. **Tension:** The state or condition resulting from muscles acting in opposition and harmony that creates the required structure, maintaining control before and/or during the chosen athletic movement.

6. **Smoothness:** The demonstration of the chosen athletic movement performed with complete control and mastery.

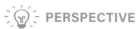
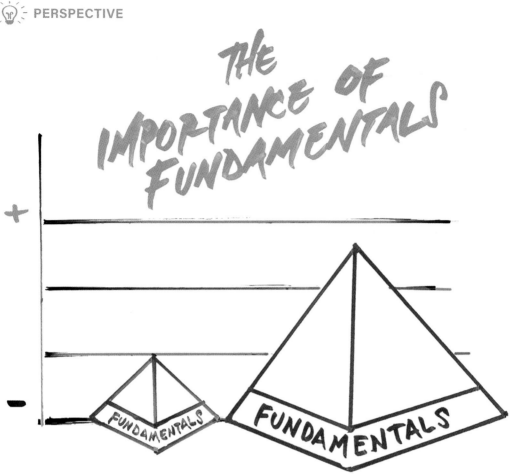

THE
IMPORTANCE OF
FUNDAMENTALS

## What does this mean?

The size and height of a pyramid is dictated by the strength and width of the base. In a similar fashion, the potential strength and skill of an athlete is dictated by their understanding and acquisition of the fundamentals.

## Why is this important?

Pushing beyond the limits of low fundamentals leads to stalled progress and/or injury.

# THE INVERTED-U THEORY

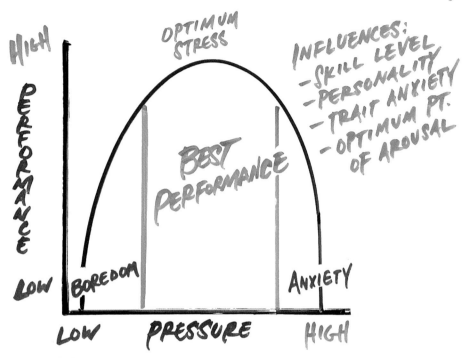

**INFLUENCES:**
- SKILL LEVEL
- PERSONALITY
- TRAIT ANXIETY
- OPTIMUM PT. OF AROUSAL

## What does this mean?

At low arousal levels, performance quality is low. Sporting performance improves as arousal levels increase, to a point. Any increase in arousal beyond the threshold point will worsen performance.

The optimal level differs from athlete to athlete based on

- Skill level
- Personality
- Trait anxiety
- Task complexity

For example, if the athlete's skill level is low, and the task is very complex, the arousal is low.

## Why is this important?

Our job as a coach is to pair the right level task with the right level athlete.

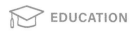

# COACHES, K.I.S.S.S. YOUR PROGRAMMING.

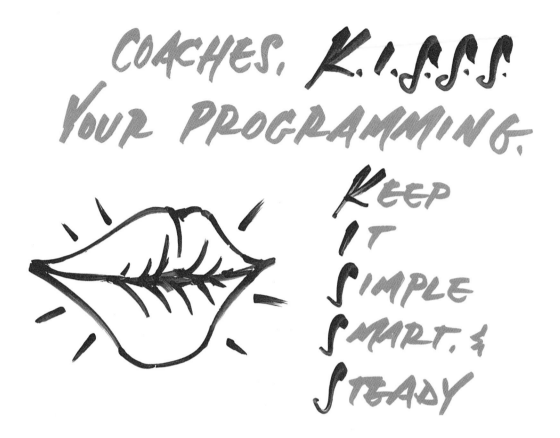

KEEP IT SIMPLE, SMART, & STEADY

## What does this mean?

When creating a program for your athletes, KEEP IT

- **Simple:** Leave out any unnecessary elements that do not benefit the goal(s) of the program.
- **Smart:** Employ a proven training methodology that is designed to accomplish the goal(s) of the program.
- **Steady:** Stick with it. Adjust as needed but understand that consistency is king.

## Why is this important?

Far too often, coaches and trainers overlook the importance of the basics. This is largely due to the athlete becoming bored with the basics. In an effort to keep the athlete engaged, the coach adds new and different exercises to keep training "fresh." Adding variety in small doses can be advantageous, but nothing beats dialing in the basics.

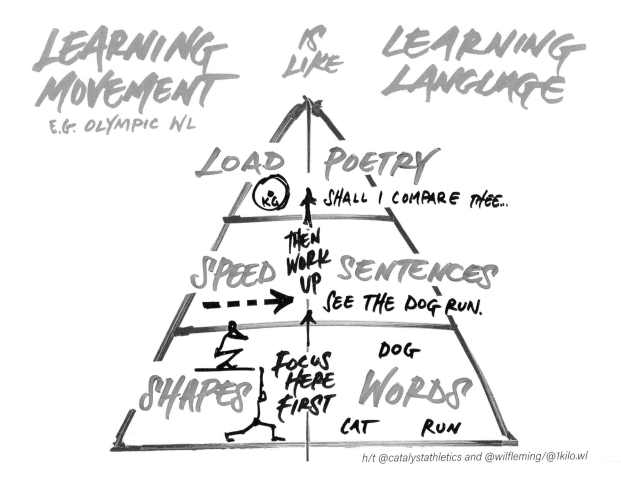

LEARNING MOVEMENT
E.G. OLYMPIC WL

IS LIKE

LEARNING LANGUAGE

LOAD — POETRY
KG SHALL I COMPARE THEE...

THEN WORK UP

SPEED — SENTENCES
SEE THE DOG RUN.

FOCUS HERE FIRST

SHAPES — DOG WORDS
CAT RUN

h/t @catalystathletics and @wilfleming/@1kilo.wl

## What does this mean?

Think about learning a language. Before you can write poetry, you need to understand grammatical structure, and before that, words.

First: Words

Then: Sentences

Finally: Poetry

## Why is this important?

There is no sense in getting wrapped up in the complexities of a movement like the clean or snatch if you cannot consistently put your body and the bar in the right position.

First: Shapes

Then: Speed

Finally: Load

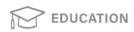 

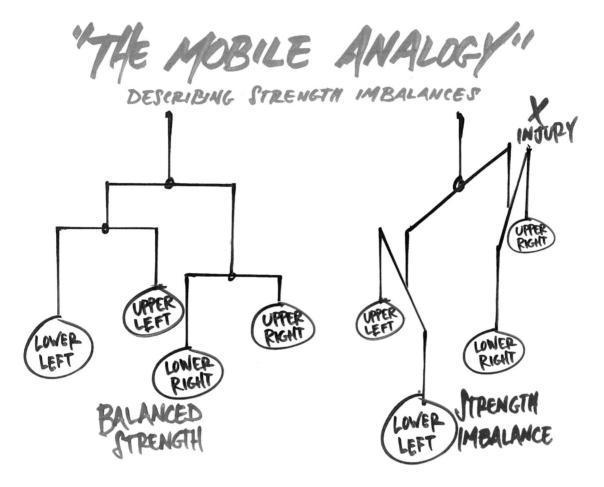

## What does this mean?

Similar to how a hanging mobile requires balance to stay in order, your body requires balance in strength to operate at a healthy level.

A simple way to correct muscle imbalances is to include unilateral strength exercises in your training. These are exercises that focus on one side of your body: single-leg squats, single-arm rows, single-leg deadlifts, and so on.

## Why is this important?

Strength imbalances eventually lead to injury due to

- Overuse of the activated muscle
- Inactive muscles
- Changing the natural path of motion for a joint

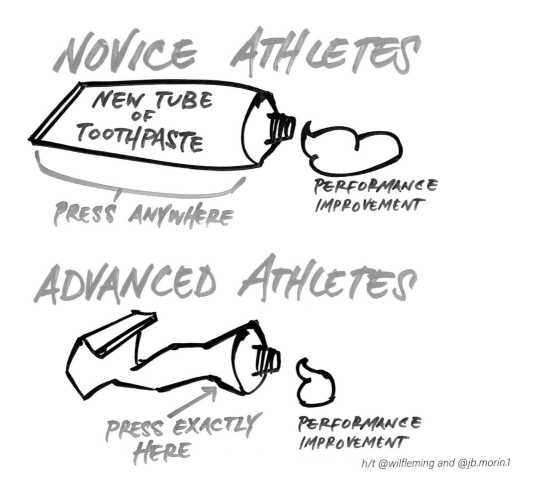

NOVICE ATHLETES

NEW TUBE OF TOOTHPASTE

PRESS ANYWHERE

PERFORMANCE IMPROVEMENT

ADVANCED ATHLETES

PRESS EXACTLY HERE

PERFORMANCE IMPROVEMENT

*h/t @wilfleming and @jb.morin.1*

## What does this mean?

Novice athletes are like a full tube of toothpaste. No matter where you press, no matter what general training they do, their performance will improve.

Advanced athletes, those who have lengthy training experience are mostly empty tubes. A coach must know exactly what type of training to prescribe, exactly where to press, in order to see noticeable improvement.

# PROGRESSION TRAINING

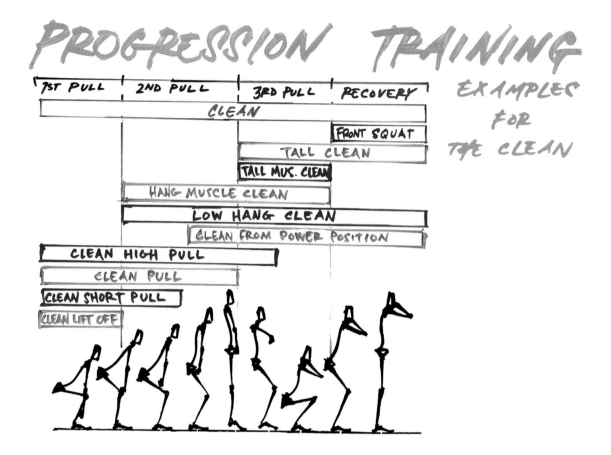

EXAMPLES FOR THE CLEAN

| 1ST PULL | 2ND PULL | 3RD PULL | RECOVERY |
|---|---|---|---|

CLEAN

FRONT SQUAT

TALL CLEAN

TALL MUS. CLEAN

HANG MUSCLE CLEAN

LOW HANG CLEAN

CLEAN FROM POWER POSITION

CLEAN HIGH PULL

CLEAN PULL

CLEAN SHORT PULL

CLEAN LIFT OFF

## When?

Refining complex movement patterns (such as the clean shown here)

## What does this mean?

Think of learning complex movement patterns like learning how to speak a long sentence. Progressions are clusters of words within the long sentence.

As the athlete takes the time to focus on the clusters of words, they strengthen their weaknesses and are able to put everything together.

## Why is this important?

When training complex movement patterns (Olympic weightlifting, gymnastics, etc.), faults will likely occur throughout the path. Using progressions allows the athlete to work on specific segments of the movement to correct faults in that component.

# PURPOSE AFFECTS ENVIRONMENT

| ┌ PURPOSE ┐ | ┌ ENVIRONMENT ┐ | | | |
|---|---|---|---|---|
| | INTENSITY | HEART RATE | FOCUS | LOAD |
| PRACTICE | VERY LOW | <65% | VERY HIGH | <60% |
| TRAINING | MOD-HIGH | 75-90% | HIGH | 75-95% |
| COMPETITION | MAX | 90-100% | SUBCONSCIOUS | 95% |

*h/t @comptrain.co*

## What does this mean?

An athlete who wants to make gains should focus more on training and practice than on competing. Training can result in big changes, whereas competing results in few gains.

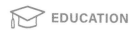
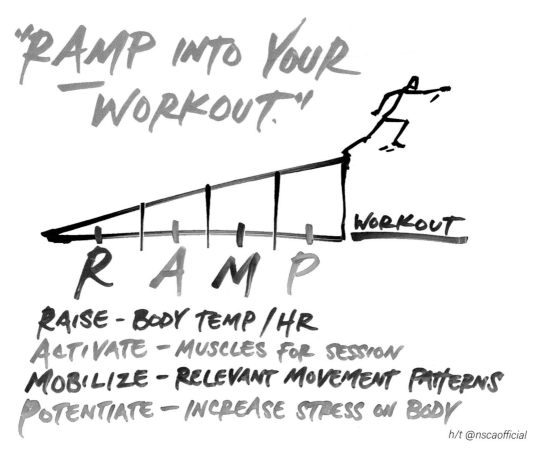

"RAMP INTO YOUR WORKOUT."

WORKOUT

R A M P

RAISE - BODY TEMP / HR
ACTIVATE - MUSCLES FOR SESSION
MOBILIZE - RELEVANT MOVEMENT PATTERNS
POTENTIATE - INCREASE STRESS ON BODY

*h/t @nscaofficial*

## What does this mean?

RAMP = Raise, Activate, Mobilize, Potentiate

- **Raise** the heart rate, respiration rate, blood flow, joint fluid viscosity using movement patterns similar to the upcoming activity.

- **Activate** the muscles that will be used for the upcoming session.

- **Mobilize** the movement patterns that will be targeted during the upcoming activity.

- **Potentiate** by using sport-specific activities that progress in intensity until the athlete is performing at the intensity required for the subsequent competition or training session.

# "RECOMMIT TO THE BASICS."

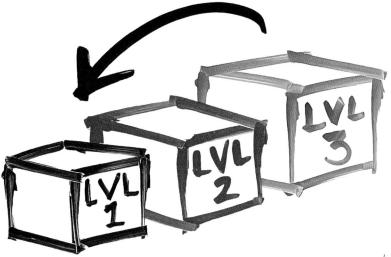

*h/t Greg Glassman*

## What does this mean?

The basics are the base or the foundation of everything else. The basics work.

## Why is this important?

If you focus on the basics and truly focus on mastering them, everything else will begin to improve. Your athletes will improve quicker, and you will gain more credibility among your peers.

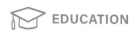

# REQUIREMENTS FOR A SUCCESSFUL LIFT

LACK CONFIDENCE/AGGRESSION

PHYSICAL ABILITY

TECHNICAL ABILITY

DON'T KNOW HOW TO MOVE

NOT STRONG ENOUGH

MENTAL FORTITUDE

## What does this mean?

When working with an athlete who keeps missing a lift, I have discovered that it comes down to three elements:

- **Physical ability:** The athlete must be physically strong enough to handle the weight of the barbell throughout the range of motion of the lift. Sometimes the athlete is simply not strong enough.

- **Technical ability:** The athlete must have a general understanding and possess the ability to move their body throughout the lift. Sometimes the athlete simply does not understand how to move.

- **Mental fortitude:** The athlete must possess the aggressive confidence to move the bar to where it needs to go. Sometimes the athlete has doubts or lacks determination.

In other words, the athlete

- Has to be strong enough
- Has to know what they're doing
- Has to want it badly enough

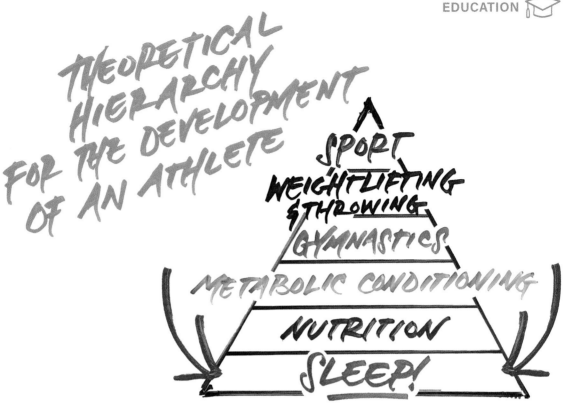

*h/t @crossfittraining Level 1 Training Guide, @ericejw163, and @nypd_crossfit*

Developed by Greg Glassman, the creator of CrossFit, the original *Theoretical Hierarchy for the Development of an Athlete* provides an overview of the elemental needs of an athlete:

- **Nutrition** is at the base because it influences metabolism; therefore, it influences the molecular foundations of muscle, bone, and the nervous system.

- **Metabolic conditioning** is next because its capacity determines the potential of strength and coordination.

- **Gymnastics** follows due to the development of body and spatial awareness. Before manipulating a barbell or kettlebell, an athlete must have a grasp on moving their body.

- **Weightlifting and throwing** follow because controlling external objects is the logical step after controlling one's body.

- **Sport** is at the peak. The foundational elements on the lower levels lead to the athlete being competitive among other people.

Eric John CF-L3 of NYPD CrossFit suggested that a person can have all the elements mastered, but without proper sleep, an athlete is at a massive disadvantage for achieving CrossFit's definition of health. Consequently, this revised version of the hierarchy has sleep as the foundational base.

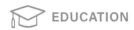 

# "SAFETY & INEFFICIENCY FAULTS"

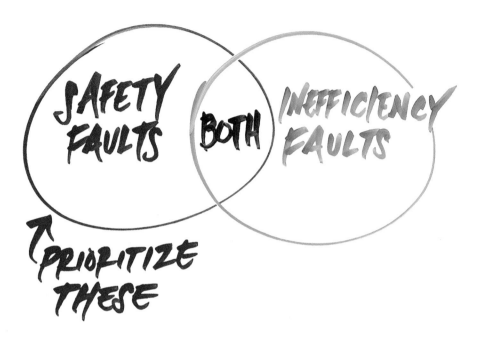

## What does this mean?

Within movement, faults fall into two broad categories:

- Safety faults
- Inefficiency faults

Some faults fall into both categories.

For example, during the first pull of the clean or snatch:

- **Safety fault:** Flexing your spine during the initial drive
- **Inefficiency fault:** Bending your arms during the initial drive
- **Safety fault *and* inefficiency fault:** Raising your hips faster than your shoulders during the initial drive

A trainer/coach should be able to correctly distinguish between the two and give priority to safety faults when correcting. As an athlete becomes more advanced, they will display fewer safety faults and more specific inefficiency faults.

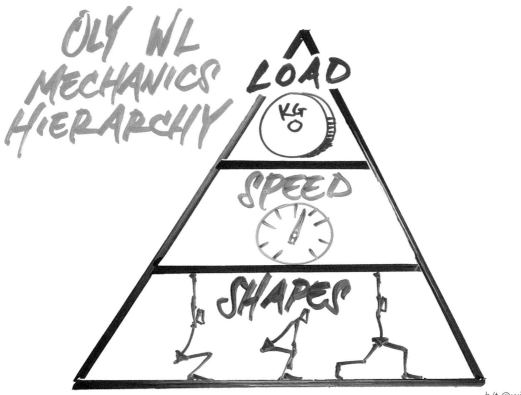

*h/t @wilfleming*

## When?

Learning or teaching Olympic weightlifting

## What does this mean?

First, you want to understand the positions or shapes that you need to achieve in the lifts so that you will have success. For example, what's a rack position? What's an overhead position? What do those positions look like and how do you move between them?

Next, move slowly between these positions and progress to moving with some speed. Getting into the positions with speed means they're recruiting bigger muscles because speed requires bigger motor units.

When you have the shapes and the speed, you can add weight. Load is the final thing to worry about.

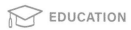 

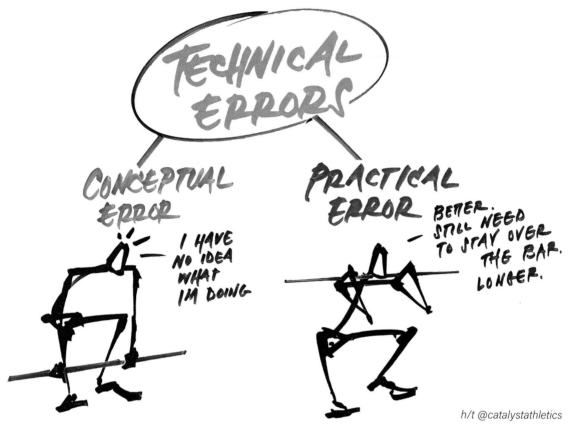

*h/t @catalystathletics*

## What does this mean?

There are two broad categories of technical errors:

- **Conceptual error:** Not knowing how to do something or having learned from improper instruction
- **Practical error:** Knowing how but improperly executing an element of the lift

The more experienced a lifter becomes, the more their errors will shift from being conceptual (they know HOW to do it) to practical (they're not executing it correctly).

Conceptual errors are normally fixed with verbal instructions and demonstration. Practical errors require more extensive intervention, including

- Drills
- Technique primers
- Standalone remedial exercises
- Modifications of lifts
- Complexes

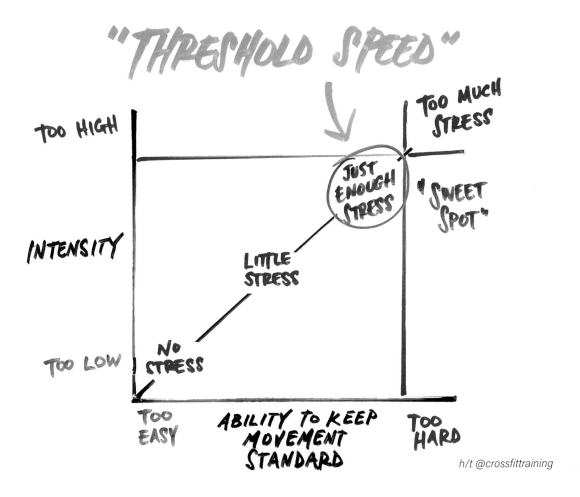

"THRESHOLD SPEED"

TOO MUCH STRESS

JUST ENOUGH STRESS

"SWEET SPOT"

TOO HIGH

INTENSITY

LITTLE STRESS

NO STRESS

TOO LOW

TOO EASY

ABILITY TO KEEP MOVEMENT STANDARD

TOO HARD

*h/t @crossfittraining*

## What does this mean?

Threshold speed is fast enough to maintain optimal intensity but slow enough to maintain movement standards.

## Why is this important?

Since intensity is a stimulus for adaptation, the higher intensity you can safely achieve while still demonstrating proper movement standards and body control, the more effective the training will be.

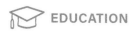
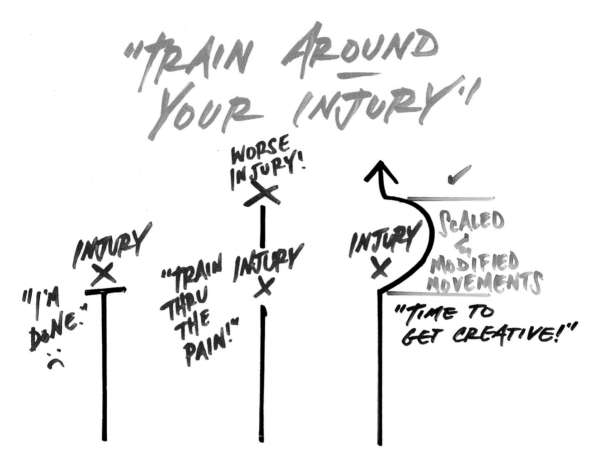

## What does this mean?

When an injury occurs, you find yourself with multiple choices.

- You can choose denial that you aren't really injured and "train through the pain," which will inevitably lead to a worse injury.

- You can choose to end your training altogether and wait until you are healed before you try to return.

- You can choose to train around your injury by following a plan that includes scaled or modified movements and specific exercises designed to strengthen the injury. This choice keeps progress rolling forward, increases your body awareness, and helps strengthen areas that may be a weakness.

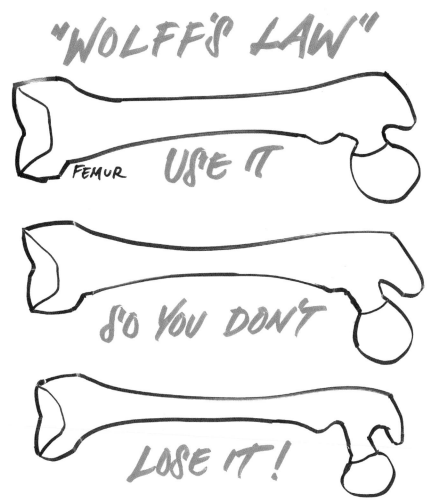

"WOLFF'S LAW"

FEMUR

USE IT

SO YOU DON'T

LOSE IT!

*h/t German anatomist and surgeon*
*Julius Wolff (1836–1902)*

Bones in a healthy person or animal adapt to the loads under which they are placed.

If loading on a particular bone increases, the bone will remodel itself over time to become stronger to resist that sort of loading.

The opposite is also true. If the loading on a bone decreases, the bone will become less dense and weaker due to the lack of the stimulus required.

# CHAPTER 6

## GRIP

# BARBELL GRIP WIDTH

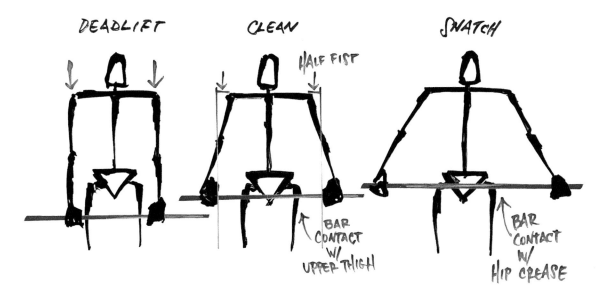

DEADLIFT     CLEAN     SNATCH

HALF FIST

BAR CONTACT W/ UPPER THIGH

BAR CONTACT W/ HIP CREASE

The following are general guidelines for grip width:

- **Deadlift grip width:** Shoulder width, hands hanging directly below shoulders, arms parallel with each other.

- **Clean grip width:** Approximately half a fist width outside the shoulders, creating a contact point for the bar on the upper thighs.

- **Snatch grip width:** Wide enough to create a contact point for the bar at the crease of the hips, just above the pubic bone.

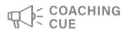
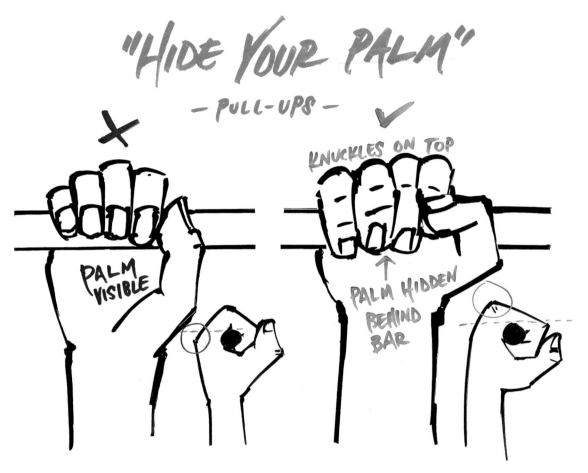

# "HIDE YOUR PALM"
## — PULL-UPS —

✗

✓

KNUCKLES ON TOP

PALM VISIBLE

↑ PALM HIDDEN BEHIND BAR

## When?

Gripping the pull-up bar

## What does this mean?

If the athlete is gripping the bar with only their fingers, the knuckles will be below the bar and the palm will be visible.

## Why is this important?

When you grip the pull-up bar with this technique, your palm is hidden behind the bar, which creates a stronger connection with the bar, improves shoulder rotation, and increases lat activation and midline tension.

# "REMEMBER YOUR RING & PINKY FINGERS"
## WHEN GRIPPING ANYTHING

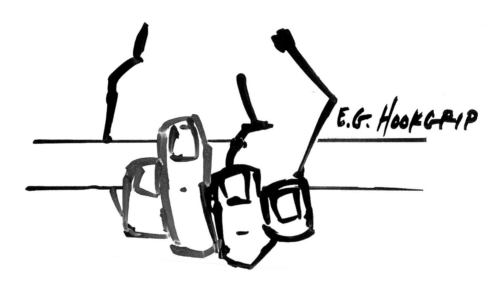

E.G. HOOKGRIP

## When?

Keeping a strong grip on an implement (bar, barbell, kettlebell, etc.)

## What does this mean?

When grip strength becomes exhausted, it's easy to focus on the index and middle finger for strength. However, don't forget about the ring and pinky fingers. A study* proves that more than 50% of grip strength comes from the pinky and ring finger.

---

*Jennifer Methot, Shrikant J. Chinchalkar, and Robert S. Richards, "Contribution of the Ulnar Digits to Grip Strength," *Plastic Surgery* 18, no. 1 (2010), https://www.ncbi.nlm.nih.gov/pmc/articles/PMC2851460/.

# CHAPTER 7

# GYMNASTICS

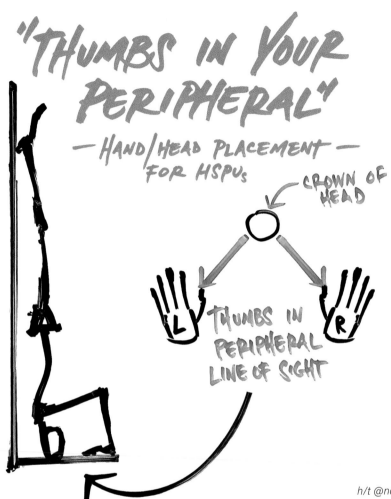

"THUMBS IN YOUR PERIPHERAL"

— HAND/HEAD PLACEMENT —
FOR HSPUs

CROWN OF HEAD

THUMBS IN PERIPHERAL LINE OF SIGHT

L    R

*h/t @no_sand_fitness*

## When?

Hand/head placement for tripod and handstand push-ups

## What does this mean?

The placement of your hands should be approximately shoulder-width and 45 degrees from the crown of your head.

If you do this correctly, you should see your thumbs in your peripheral vision.

## Why is this important?

The bottom of a handstand push-up should be a strong tripod position with the crown of the head and both hands making up the three points of contact.

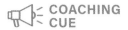
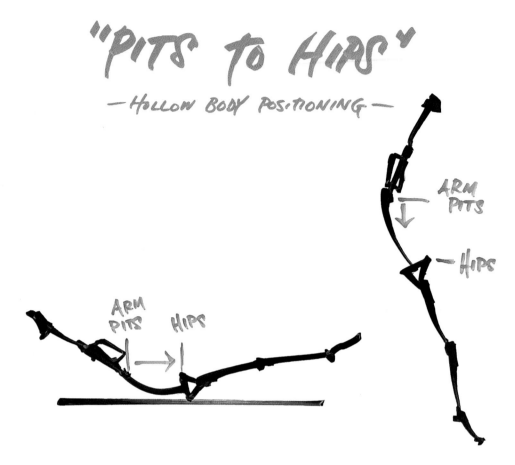

*"PITS TO HIPS"*

— HOLLOW BODY POSITIONING —

ARM PITS

HIPS

ARM PITS   HIPS

## When?

Hollow body position

## What does this mean?

A key to setting the hollow position is to engage your abdominal muscles to pull your armpits toward your hips.

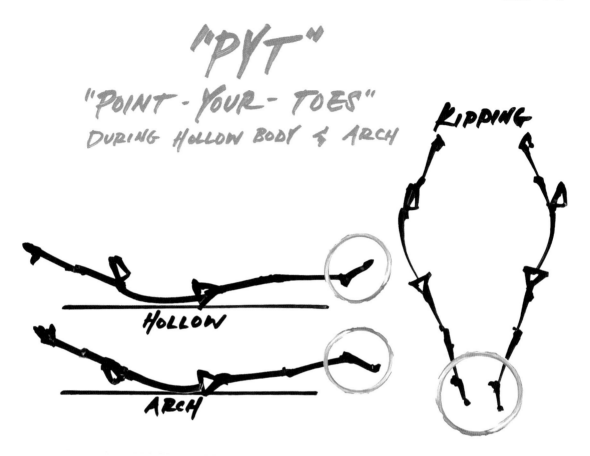

"PYT"
"POINT - YOUR - TOES"
DURING HOLLOW BODY & ARCH

KIPPING

HOLLOW

ARCH

### When?
Hollow body and arch movements, such as kipping movements (pull-ups, muscle-ups, toes-to-bar, etc.)

### What does this mean?
During efficient kipping movements, the body moves through hollow body and arch positions. This allows you to create tension throughout the body that can be used as power to drive through a movement pattern (e.g., a pull-up). Pointing the toes helps create tension by activating muscles in the lower body.

### Why is this important?
Pointing your toes helps you maximize your power potential.

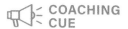

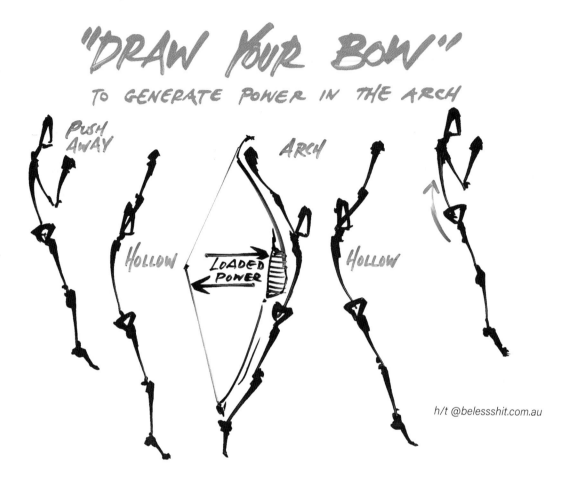

"DRAW YOUR BOW"
TO GENERATE POWER IN THE ARCH

PUSH AWAY · ARCH · HOLLOW · LOADED POWER · HOLLOW

h/t @belessshit.com.au

## When?

Kipping movements—pull-ups and muscle-ups

## What does this mean?

To generate power, especially when linking together kipping pull-ups and bar muscle-ups, move from a hollow position into an arch position. The arch position should resemble a bow being drawn, with the upper and lower tips being pulled back. Use this energy to drive back into the hollow position and into your next rep.

# KIPPING PULL-UP

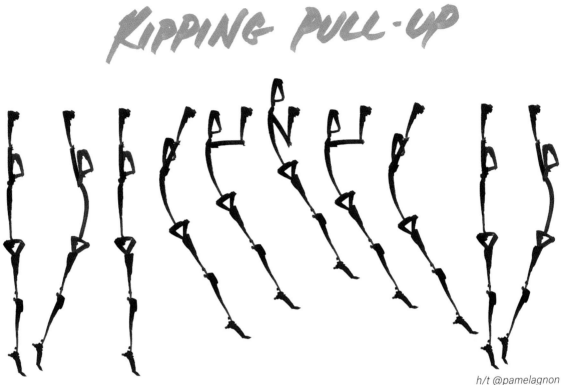

*h/t @pamelagnon*

## Prerequisites

You should be able to do three to six strict pull-ups *before* adding momentum. Kipping is *not* a substitute for the inability to do a strict movement.

## Setup:

- Hands just outside shoulder width
- Full grip on the bar

## Movement:

- Start in a hanging position with your arms extended.
- Use your shoulders to initiate a swing.
- Alternate between arched and hollow positions.
- Drive your hips toward the bar while in the hollow position.
- At the same time, push down on the bar with straight arms.
- Rapidly extend your hips and then pull with your arms.
- Pull until your chin is higher than the bar.
- Initiate descent by pushing away from the bar.

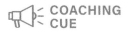
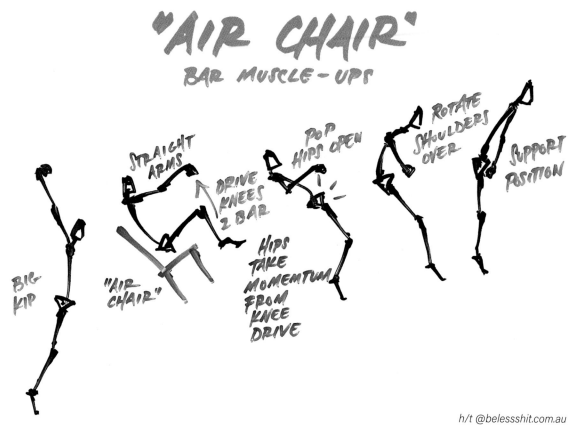

*"AIR CHAIR"*

*BAR MUSCLE-UPS*

BIG KIP

"AIR CHAIR"

STRAIGHT ARMS

DRIVE KNEES 2 BAR

HIPS TAKE MOMEMTUM FROM KNEE DRIVE

POP HIPS OPEN

ROTATE SHOULDERS OVER

SUPPORT POSITION

*h/t @belessshit.com.au*

## When?

Bar muscle-ups

## What does this mean?

Think about the position you take when you are reclined in a chair: slight knee and hip flexion. During the kip, try to establish this position while driving your knees toward the bar. Once you reach approximately a femur's length away from the bar, kick against the air and stand up out of your chair. Use the momentum created from the explosive hip and knee extension toward your upper body.

# "FALL LIKE A FEATHER"

### ON DOWNWARD PHASE OF KIPPING RING MUP

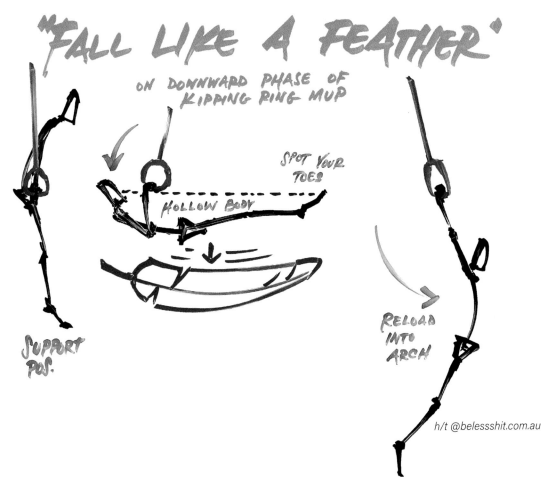

SPOT YOUR TOES

HOLLOW BODY

SUPPORT POS.

RELOAD INTO ARCH

*h/t @belessshit.com.au*

## When?

On the downward phase of the ring muscle-up

## What does this mean?

From the support position, initiate the downward phase by falling back into a hollow body position. Lengthen your body and spot your toes on the descent, so you're shaped similarly to a feather.

## Why is this important?

The tension you maintain through the hollow position generates power into your arch at the bottom and allows you to reload into your next rep.

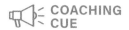
# "KNEES TO THE BAR"
## BAR MUSCLE-UPS

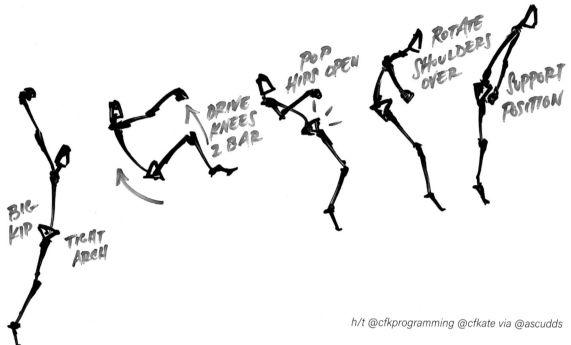

BIG KIP

TIGHT ARCH

DRIVE KNEES 2 BAR

POP HIPS OPEN

ROTATE SHOULDERS OVER

SUPPORT POSITION

*h/t @cfkprogramming @cfkate via @ascudds*

## When?

Bar muscle-ups

## What does this mean?

During the drive, focus on getting your knees to the bar before you transition over. Carry this momentum through an explosive hip extension to drive your body up and over.

# "MERMAID SUIT"

## — KIPPING MOVEMENTS E.G. RING MUSCLE-UPS

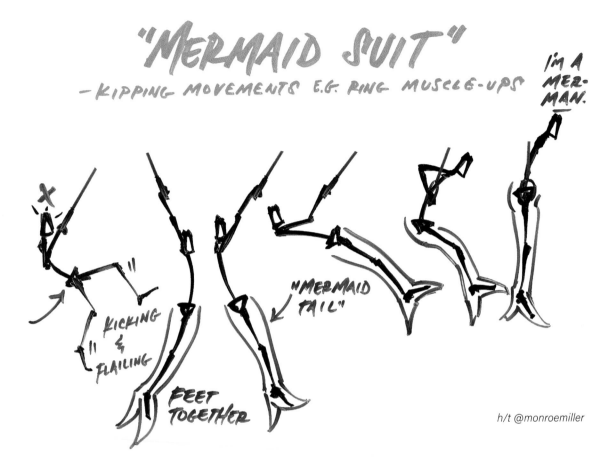

I'M A MER-MAN.

X

KICKING & FLAILING

"MERMAID TAIL"

FEET TOGETHER

h/t @monroemiller

## When?

Kipping movements, especially ring muscle-ups

## What does this mean?

A mermaid has one tail, not two legs. During kipping gymnastics movements, keep your legs together to generate power from your lower body.

## Why is this important?

You can generate more power when your legs work together rather than independently.

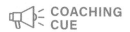
# "PUSH THE RINGS FORWARD"
## DURING RING MUP

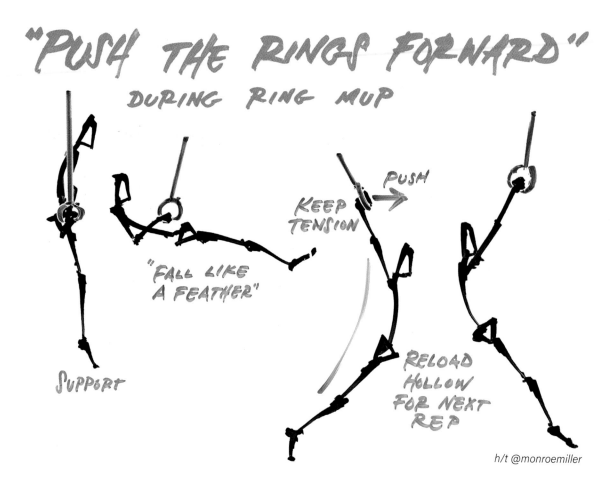

SUPPORT

"FALL LIKE A FEATHER"

KEEP TENSION

PUSH

RELOAD HOLLOW FOR NEXT REP

*h/t @monroemiller*

### When?
Kipping ring muscle-ups

### What does this mean?
During the kipping ring muscle-up, it's crucial to maintain tension through your body by using the hollow and arch positions. Keep the tension connected from the body and through the rings by pushing them forward during the arch position of the kip.

### Why is this important?
Doing this helps you reload into the hollow position and drive into your next rep.

# "TRUCKER HORN"
## (OR TRAIN)

### "HONK-HHHHONK" — PULL-UP ELBOW POSITION —

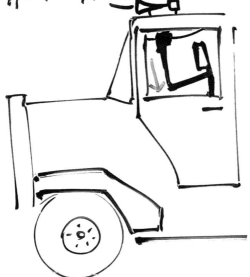

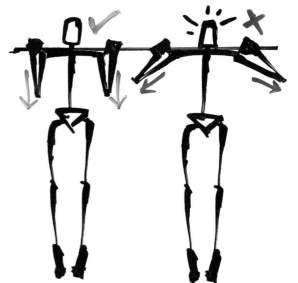

*h/t @coach_birdy via @birdbox_coaching/@thegymnasticscourse*

## When?

Elbow position during the pull-up

## What does this mean?

When a truck driver or train driver honks their horn, they pull down (not out) on a rope above their head. During the pull-up, drive the elbows down, not out.

## Why is this important?

During the pull-up, your shoulder position should be externally rotated because it's both safer for the joint and engages more of your lats.

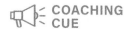
COACHING CUE

# "HINGE INTO YOUR PISTOL"

## TO LEARN OR WARM-UP FOR PISTOLS

BALANCE ON ONE FOOT

BEND OVER AND GRAB FREE FOOT

HINGE YOUR BODY AROUND YOUR KNEE

HIP CREASE BELOW TOP OF KNEE

NOW REVERSE

## When?

Learning the pistol squat

## What does this mean?

Try this technique when learning or warming up for your pistol squats:

1. Stand on one foot, with the other foot barely off the ground.

2. Bend over and grab your free foot with the hand on the same side.

3. Hinging around your knee on the support leg, send your hips back and down while still holding your foot and keeping your knee straight.

4. Reverse the steps to stand.

# "STAY IN THE PHONE BOOTH"
## DURING KIPPING TOES 2 BAR

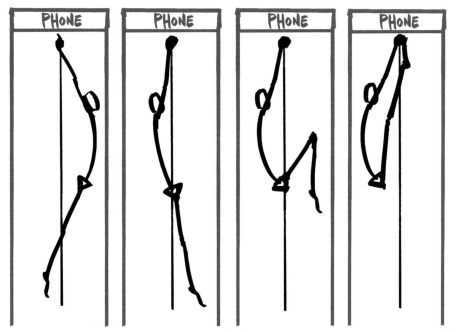

*h/t @thegymnasticscourse coach @chuckbennington*

## When?

Kipping toes to bar

## What does this mean?

Imagine you are moving in a phone booth and have to keep from hitting the walls. Stay tight on the "toe tap" to the bar and cycle down into the next rep. Additionally, keep even on each side of the bar in the hollow and arch positions.

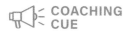

COACHING
CUE

# "PULL THE BAR DOWN"
## — STRICT PULL-UPS —

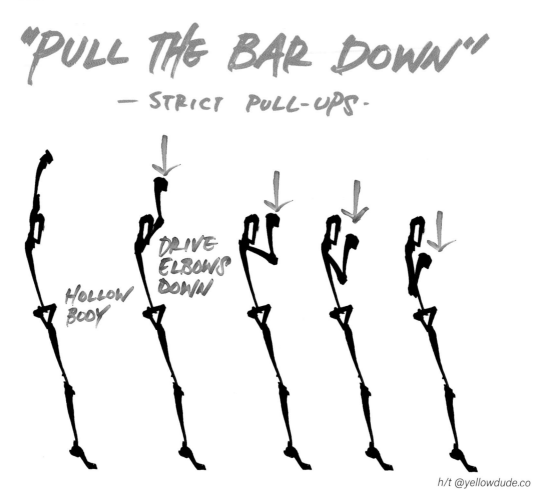

*h/t @yellowdude.co*

### When?

Strict pull-ups

### What does this mean?

Pull yourself up by visualizing that you're pulling the bar down. Initiate the pull-up by retracting your shoulders and then drive your elbows down to pull yourself up.

Similar to the deadlift and push-up cue "push the Earth away," sometimes changing your perspective of the movement sequence can help things click.

# SCALING GYMNASTICS MOVEMENTS

## DELOAD ATHLETE = + FULL ROM

E.G. HSPU

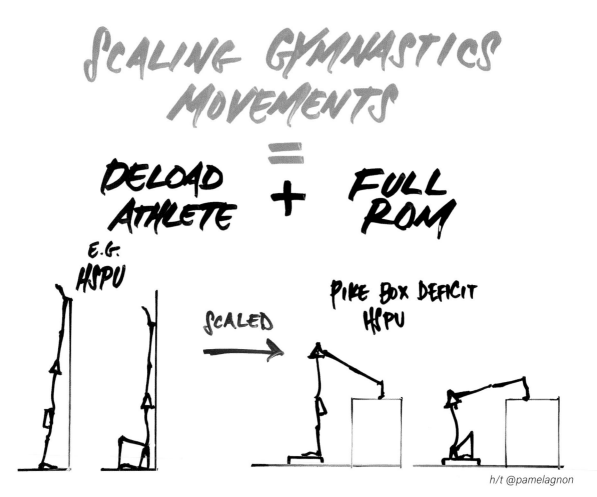

SCALED

PIKE BOX DEFICIT HSPU

h/t @pamelagnon

## What does this mean?

The value in movement is found in strength throughout a full range of motion. You cannot build strength in a full range of motion if you cannot safely move through a full range of motion.

If a gymnastics movement is too difficult, rather than shorten the range of motion, deload the movement and build strength through the full range of motion. As strength increases, you can reintroduce load.

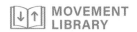
# "THE BURPEE"

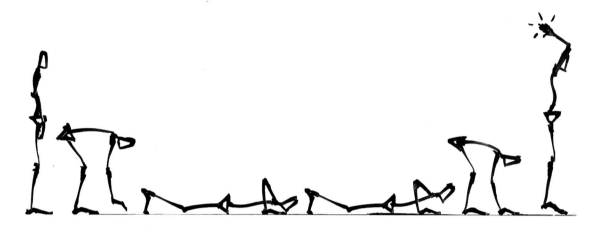

## Points of Performance

- Place your hands on the ground, shoulder width apart.

- Jump to the push-up position.

- Lower your chest and thighs to the ground.

- Push up and jump your feet up to your hands.

- Jump vertically with full hip and knee extension while extending your arms overhead.

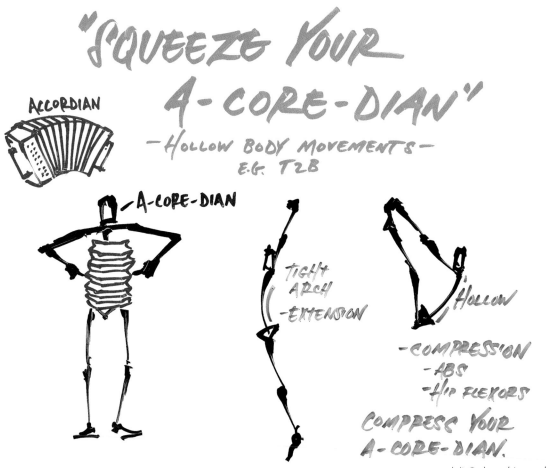

"SQUEEZE YOUR
A-CORE-DIAN"
— HOLLOW BODY MOVEMENTS —
E.G. T2B

ACCORDIAN

A-CORE-DIAN

TIGHT
ARCH
-EXTENSION

HOLLOW

-COMPRESSION
-ABS
-HIP FLEXORS

COMPRESS YOUR
A-CORE-DIAN.

h/t @clcoachtocoach

## When?

Hollow body movements (e.g., toes-to-bar)

## What does this mean?

Your core expands and compresses similar to an accordion. It flexes and extends. During gymnastic movements (hollow body, arch, etc.), use your core for what it was designed to do, and you will become more efficient.

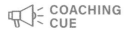

# COACHING CUE

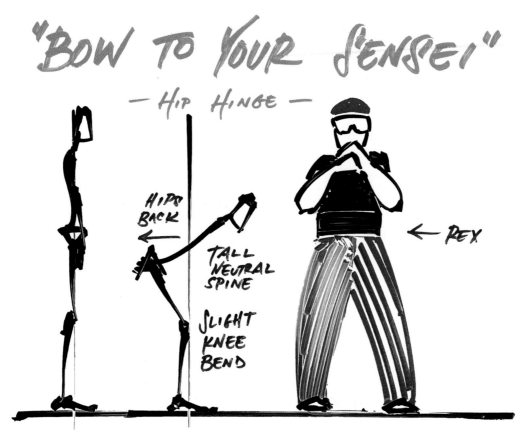

## "BOW TO YOUR SENSEI"
### — HIP HINGE —

HIPS BACK

TALL NEUTRAL SPINE

SLIGHT KNEE BEND

← REX

## When?

Hinge movements

## What does this mean?

Similar to bowing to your "sensei" (i.e., the barbell), show respect and don't be a slouch.

The hinge is essentially a bow. Keep your spine tall and your chest proud, send your hips back, and bend your knees without moving them forward.

## Why is this important?

Although the hinge movement is centered around the hips, a tall spine and engaged musculature of the torso is crucial to its effectiveness.

# "DOUBLE STRING"
## FOR HIP HINGE

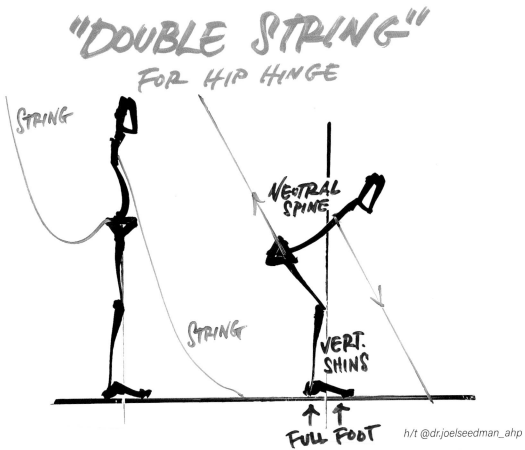

STRING

STRING

NEUTRAL SPINE

VERT. SHINS

FULL FOOT

*h/t @dr.joelseedman_ahp*

## When?

Hip hinge

## What does this mean?

Imagine you have a string pulling your chest toward the floor and another string pulling your hips up and back toward the ceiling.

## Why is this important?

Understanding the sequence of movement for the hip hinge builds body awareness and enables you to apply this skill to other movements.

## Points of performance:

- Neutral spine
- Slight bend in your knees
- Vertical shins
- Full foot pressure

# CHAPTER ⑧

## KETTLEBELLS

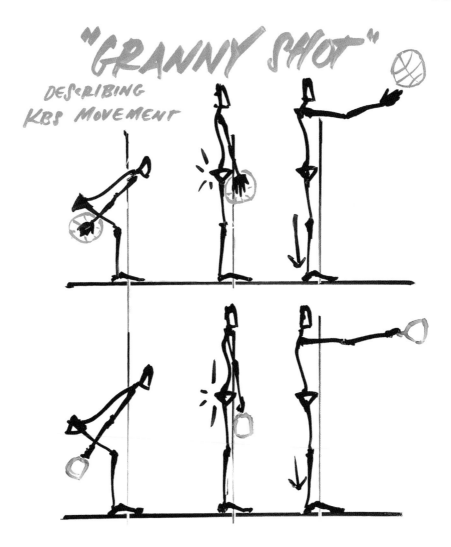

"GRANNY SHOT"
DESCRIBING
KBS MOVEMENT

## When?

Describing the kettlebell swing movement

## What does this mean?

Similar to a "granny shot" in basketball, the movement of the kettlebell swing is a hip hinge into hip and knee extension.

The stance is approximately shoulder-width apart. Your hips go back and your knees bend, but your shins stay vertical. The kettlebell swing is powered by the hips driving open as you stand tall with full extension of your hips and knees.

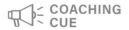

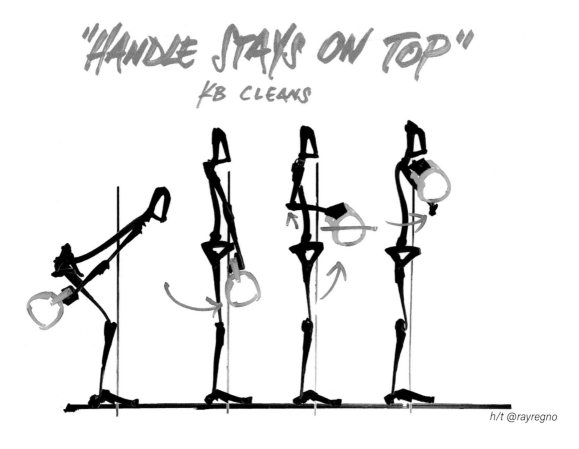

"HANDLE STAYS ON TOP"
KB CLEANS

*h/t @rayregno*

## When?

Kettlebell clean

## What does this mean?

A common error with the KB clean is the bell of the kettlebell flipping above the handle during the turnover. Instead, keep the handle above the center of mass of the bell throughout the clean.

## Why is this important?

Keeping the handle above the center of mass prevents the bell from banging on the back of your forearm during the receive. Your receive will be smooth and efficient.

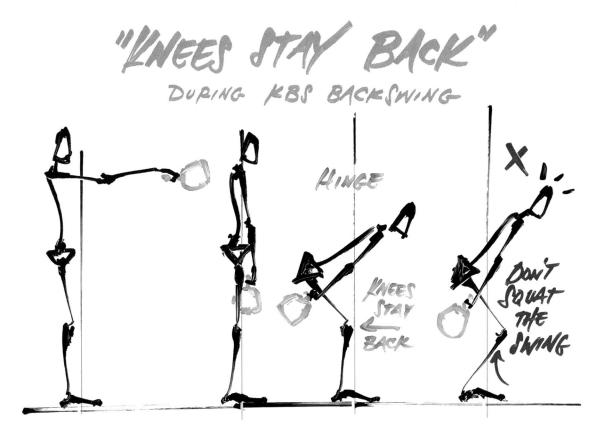

# "KNEES STAY BACK"
## DURING KBS BACKSWING

HINGE

KNEES
STAY
← BACK

✗

DON'T
SQUAT
THE
SWING

### When?
During the backswing of the kettlebell swing

### What does this mean?
As the forearms make contact with the hips during the backswing of the kettlebell swing, receive the kettlebell in a hinge. The hinge movement pattern brings the shoulders forward, hips back, and keeps the shins vertical.

### Why is this important?
Using this technique safely loads the posterior chain with power for the next swing.

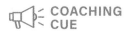
# "NEWSPAPER IN THE ARMPIT"
## FOR KB CLEANS

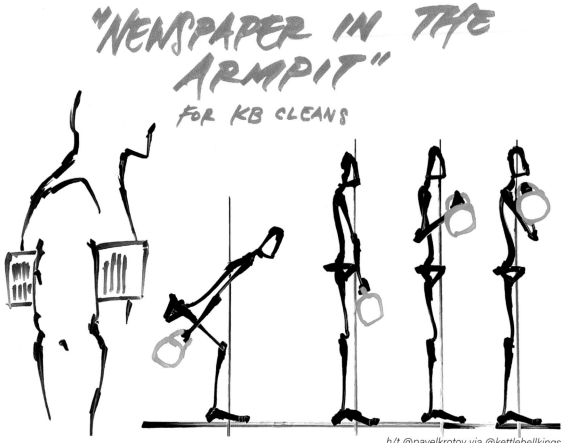

*h/t @pavelkrotov via @kettlebellkings*

## When?

Kettlebell cleans

## What does this mean?

A common error for the single-arm kettlebell clean is casting the KB too far out in front or looping the kettlebell path. This results in the KB landing with a bang on your forearm. Instead, keep your upper arm close to your body, as if you're pinching a newspaper in your armpit.

## Why is this important?

Keeping your "cleaning arm" close to the rib cage throughout the entire motion helps guide the path of the kettlebell.

# "DRIVE OFF-ARM FORWARD"
## - SINGLE-ARM OH PRESS -

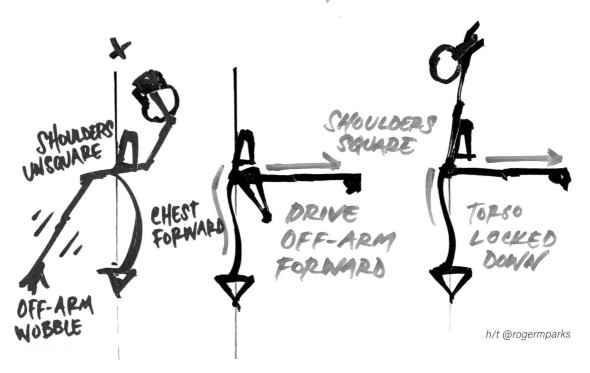

SHOULDERS UNSQUARE

CHEST FORWARD

OFF-ARM WOBBLE

SHOULDERS SQUARE

DRIVE OFF-ARM FORWARD

SHOULDERS SQUARE

TORSO LOCKED DOWN

*h/t @rogermparks*

## When?

Single arm overhead press

## What does this mean?

Pushing your chest forward during the press can make up for deficits in shoulder motion. However, it can also strain your back and make your press weaker.

If you have the tendency to push your chest forward, instead, drive your nonworking arm forward to square your shoulders.

## Why is this important?

Moving back slightly is acceptable but pushing your chest forward causes problems in most cases. Driving your arm forward mitigates the potential for straining your back.

# CHAPTER ⑨

## MISCELLANEOUS

# "HANDS ABOVE HEAD"
## — START OF BROAD JUMP —

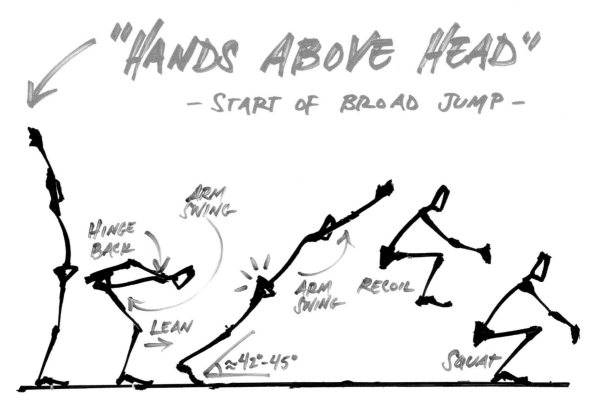

HINGE BACK

ARM SWING

LEAN

ARM SWING

≈ 42° - 45°

RECOIL

SQUAT

## When?
Starting a broad jump

## What does this mean?
A strong forward arm swing can help carry the momentum generated by the lower body. Get the most out of it by initiating the movement by starting with the hands above the head, moving into a strong back swing, and bringing the hands above the head again as you fully extend your hips and knees.

## Why is this important?
Arms play a massive role in the distance of the broad jump. A better start will lead to a better finish.

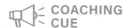

COACHING
CUE

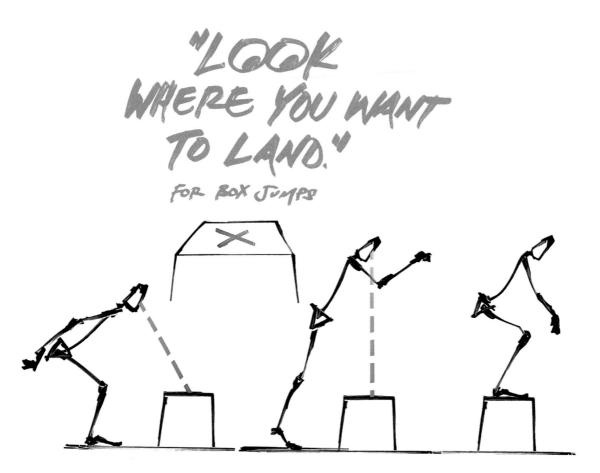

## When?

Box jumps

## What does this mean?

When shooting a basketball, look where you want the ball to go.

When throwing a football, look where you want the pass to go.

When pitching a baseball, look where you want the ball to go.

Similar to other sports, when doing box jumps, keep your focus where you want to land.

# "TRIPLE EXTENSION"
## - EXTENSION THROUGH HIP, KNEE, ANKLE

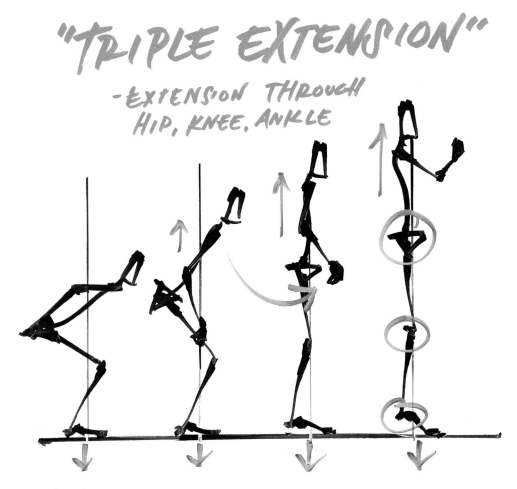

## When?
Countless athletic movements

## What does this mean?
Triple extension refers to the explosive generation of power produced by the simultaneous extension of the hips, knees, and ankles.

## Why is this important?
The better you understand how the hips, knees, and ankles work together to create power, the easier it will be to transfer this skill across multiple explosive, athletic movements.

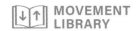
# "LIFT → LAP → LOVE → LAUNCH"

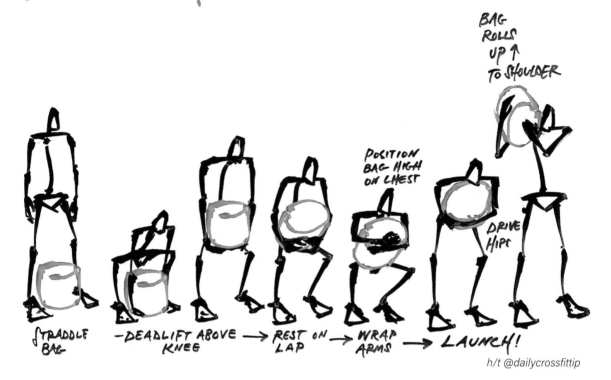

BAG ROLLS UP ↑ TO SHOULDER

POSITION BAG HIGH ON CHEST

DRIVE HIPS

STRADDLE BAG — DEADLIFT ABOVE KNEE → REST ON LAP → WRAP ARMS → LAUNCH!

*h/t @dailycrossfittip*

## When?

Strongman sandbag cleans

## What does this mean?

**Lift:** Deadlift the sandbag to above your knees.

**Lap:** Set the sandbag down on your lap.

**Love:** Hug the sandbag and position it high on your chest.

**Launch:** Drive your hips up and open and roll the sandbag up your chest to your shoulder.

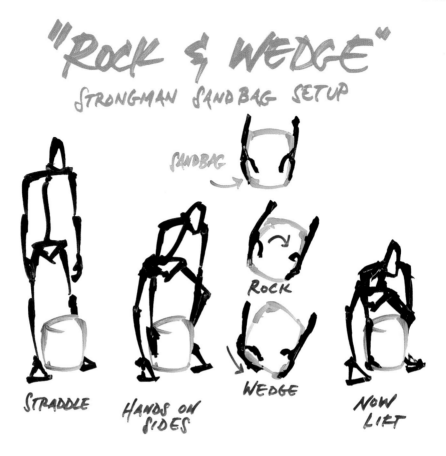

# "ROCK & WEDGE"
## STRONGMAN SANDBAG SETUP

SANDBAG

ROCK

WEDGE

STRADDLE

HANDS ON SIDES

NOW LIFT

## When?

Picking up a strongman sandbag

## What does this mean?

During the setup, take an approximate shoulder-width stance with your feet on either side of the sandbag.

Place your hands on either side of the sandbag.

Rock the sandbag back and forth. With each rock, wedge your fingertips underneath the sandbag until you have a firm grip.

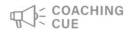
# "BOTTOM HEMISPHERE"
## HAND PLACEMENT FOR WALL BALLS

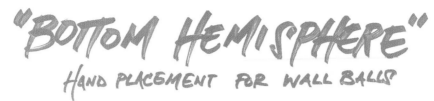

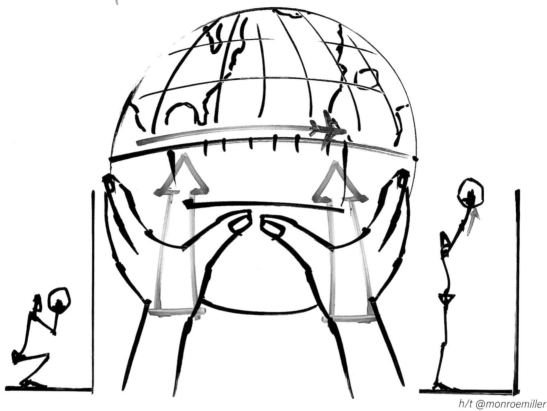

*h/t @monroemiller*

## When?

Hand position during wall balls

## What does this mean?

Whenever you're shooting or receiving a medicine ball, try to keep your hands on the bottom hemisphere of the ball.

## Why is this important?

Holding the ball on the bottom leads to a more efficient transfer of power up and into the ball.

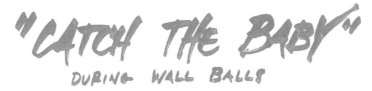

# "CATCH THE BABY"
## DURING WALL BALLS

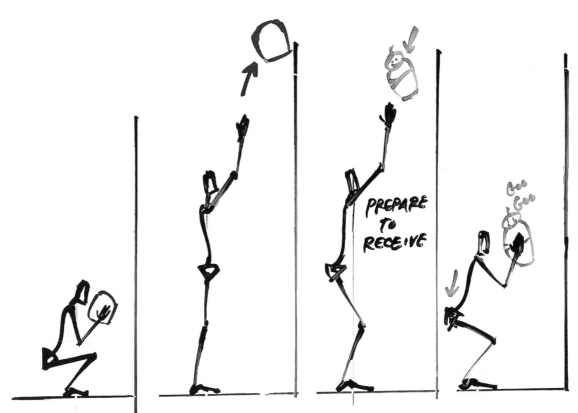

PREPARE
TO
RECEIVE

Goo Goo

### When?
Wall balls

### What does this mean?
Prepare for the impact of the wall ball by slightly bending your arms and legs. As the ball falls back down, catch the ball softly and smoothly transition into the squat.

### Why is this important?
For a movement that typically has higher reps, like wall balls, it's important to have a smooth transition of receiving the ball and leading into the squat.

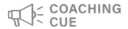
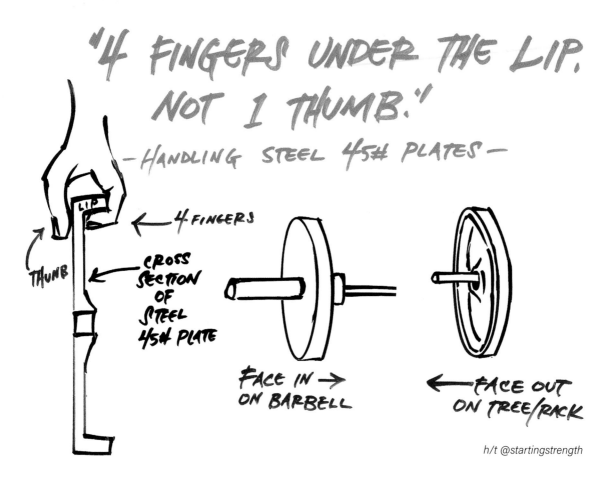

"4 FINGERS UNDER THE LIP,
NOT 1 THUMB."

— HANDLING STEEL 45# PLATES —

THUMB

LIP

← 4 FINGERS

CROSS
SECTION
OF
STEEL
45# PLATE

FACE IN →
ON BARBELL

← FACE OUT
ON TREE/RACK

*h/t @startingstrength*

## When?

Handling steel 45-pound plates

## What does this mean?

Believe it or not, there is a safe way to handle steel 45-pound plates. The plates normally have a face and a backside. The face of the plate has a lip that runs around the entire edge of the plate. This is also the side that has lettering or numbers. The backside is entirely smooth and flat.

Maneuver these plates so your four fingers grab the lip of the plate, so the plate faces out. Your thumb is on the smooth backside. This grip allows you to have the best hold on the plate when loading and unloading a barbell.

# "IT'S ALL IN THE HIPS."
## – CHUBBS PETERSON

STRONGMAN

SNATCHES

CLEANS

VIOLENT HIP EXTENSION

SPRINTS

KIPPING

JUMPING

KETTLEBELL

SQUATS

## What does this mean?

The glutes and hamstring muscle groups are the primary extensors of the hip joint. They're responsible for the violent extension of the hip joint that's required in nearly every explosive movement performed in athletics and conditioning.

## Why is this important?

When introducing a new movement to an athlete, referencing commonalities from other familiar movements may help them transfer the skills necessary to be successful.

For programs that focus on work capacity across broad time and modal domains, no other skill transfers to more movements than "violent hip extension."

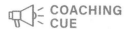
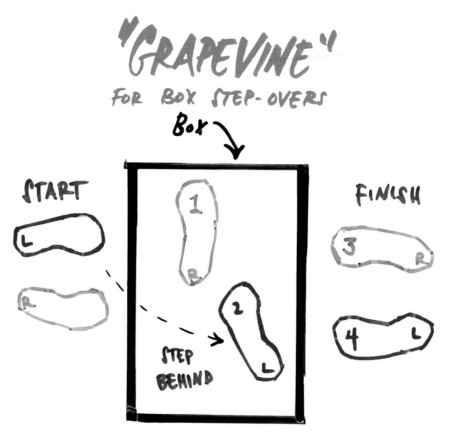

## When?

Box step-overs

## What does this mean?

Doing the grapevine step during box step-overs is an efficient method for meeting the standard of both feet touching the top of the box, as well as minimizing the number of steps needed.

## Why is this important?

By placing your second foot behind the first foot you used to step up, you are in the position to easily step down without changing direction on the floor. You're ready for the next rep!

# "HANDS TO POCKETS"
## — CROSSOVER JUMPS —

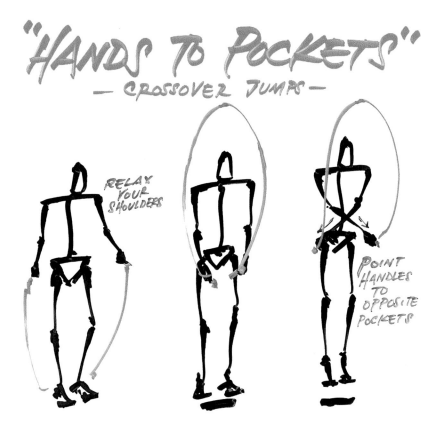

RELAX YOUR SHOULDERS

POINT HANDLES TO OPPOSITE POCKETS

*h/t @elite_srs*

### When?

Crossover jumps when jumping rope

### What does this mean?

Three cues to remember when attempting crossovers:

1.  **Relax your shoulders:** Keeping your shoulders down and relaxed reduces the amount of movement in your upper body (resulting in less wasted energy) and keeps your hands close to your hips.

2.  **Point your handles**: By pointing your handles down to your opposite pockets ("hands to pockets"), you keep your hands close to your body and reduce the amount of time it takes to transition from a cross to a standard jump.

3.  **Cross second:** Let your first rotation be a standard jump and the second rotation be your cross. This enables you to focus on your jump form as you take off and streamlines your jumps to help you start performing your double under crosses unbroken!

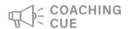
# "HAT TO POCKETS"
## SKIERG DRIVE

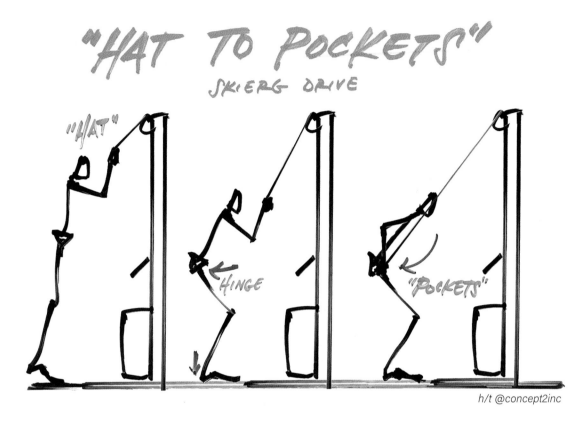

"HAT"

HINGE

"POCKETS"

h/t @concept2inc

## When?

Using the Concept2 SkiErg drive

## What does this mean?

Initiate the catch with your arms bent at 90° and your hands slightly above eye level (your hat).

During the drive, your hands move to your hips (your "pockets").

Use your core to initiate the drive. Hinge at your hips before bending your knees to drive the handles down.

After each pull, your knees are bent, and your hands are by your hips. Your arms do not fully extend.

## Why is this important?

Following an efficient movement sequence provides a balance between generating power and saving energy.

# "HEAVY IN THE HAND, FAST IN THE FEET."

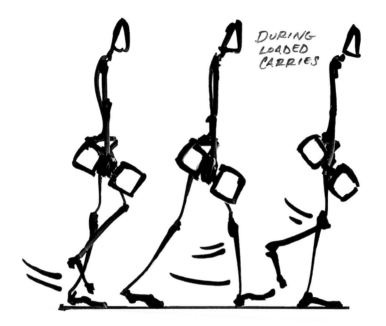

DURING LOADED CARRIES

*h/t @invictusboston*

### When?

Loaded carries like the farmer's carry or sandbag carry

### What does this mean?

Move your feet as fast as you can while controlling the load during carries.

People often make the mistake of moving slowly because the weight feels heavy in their hands when it's actually relatively light for their legs to move. Challenge yourself to pick up the pace with your feet, and you'll incur less fatigue on your grip.

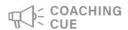

# "HOP ON YOUR SURFBOARD"
## BAR-FACING BURPEES

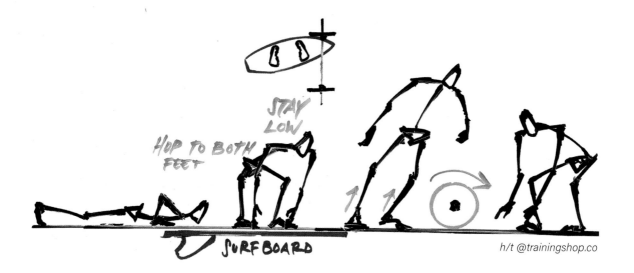

h/t @trainingshop.co

## When?

Bar-facing burpees

## What does this mean?

When doing a bar-facing burpee, it should look like you're trying to hop onto a surfboard; both feet landing at the same time and keeping your center of gravity low.

# "KNEE OVER FOOT"
## ON THE AIR BIKE

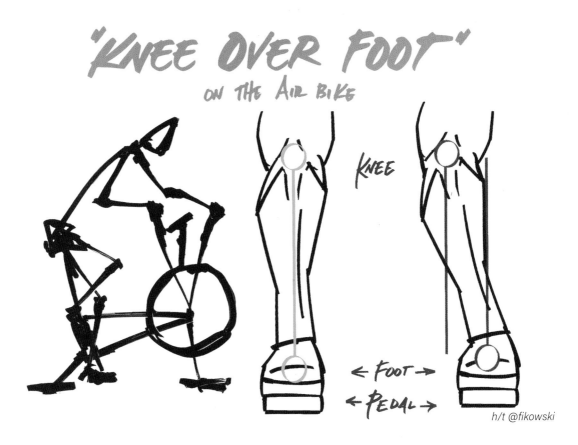

KNEE

← FOOT →
← PEDAL →

h/t @fikowski

### When?

Using the air bike

### What does this mean?

Maintaining the knee drive directly over the foot ensures the power is going into the pedal.

### Why is this important?

Maintaining this alignment keeps the transfer of power from the hip to the pedal as efficient as possible.

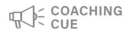

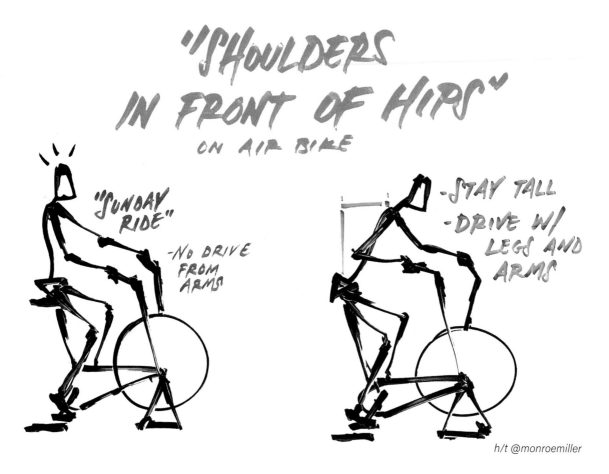

"SHOULDERS IN FRONT OF HIPS"
ON AIR BIKE

"SUNDAY RIDE"

-NO DRIVE FROM ARMS

-STAY TALL
-DRIVE W/ LEGS AND ARMS

*h/t @monroemiller*

## When?

Air bike

## What does this mean?

When you're riding the bike, sit tall and lean forward so your shoulders are positioned ahead of your hips. This puts you in a more efficient position to keep your airway open and use your arms and your legs together to crank on the bike.

# "KNEES EXTEND"
## GHD SIT-UP ASCENT

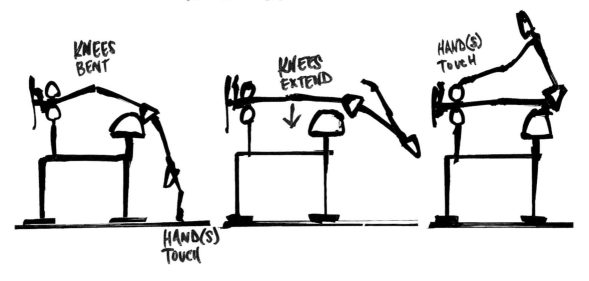

### When?
During the ascent on the GHD sit-up

### What does this mean?
As your torso descends, your knees should remain slightly bent. You initiate the ascent by aggressively extending your knees.

### Why is this important?
The focus of the GHD sit-up is commonly on flexion and extension of the core. However, the legs provide a powerful initial drive to send the wave of contraction into motion. Using the legs makes this movement more efficient.

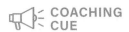
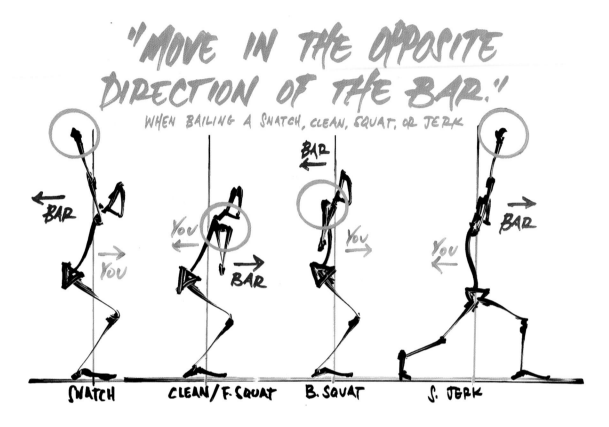

"MOVE IN THE OPPOSITE DIRECTION OF THE BAR."

WHEN BAILING A SNATCH, CLEAN, SQUAT, OR JERK

SNATCH    CLEAN / F. SQUAT    B. SQUAT    S. JERK

## When?

Bailing from a snatch, clean, squat variation, or jerk

## What does this mean?

If you lose control of a lift, don't have the strength to complete the lift, or feel you're about to injure yourself, BAIL. Do not try to save it. Get out of the way and let the bar fall to the ground.

When bailing a lift, simply move in the opposite direction of the bar to get out of the way:

- If you lose control of the lift when the bar is in front of your midline, move back to get out of the way.

- If you lose control of the lift when the bar is behind your midline, move forward to get out of the way.

## Why is this important?

Bailing from a lift is an eventual necessity during training. Doing so improperly may cause injury.

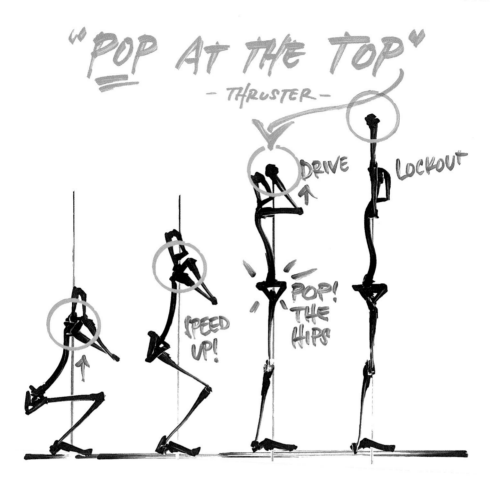

## When?

Thruster

## What does this mean?

As you drive out of the bottom of the thruster, aggressively extend your hips (POP!) to transfer power through the front rack and into the push press.

Think of the front rack as a launch pad for the barbell. The momentum from the front squat drives seamlessly into pressing the bar overhead.

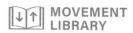

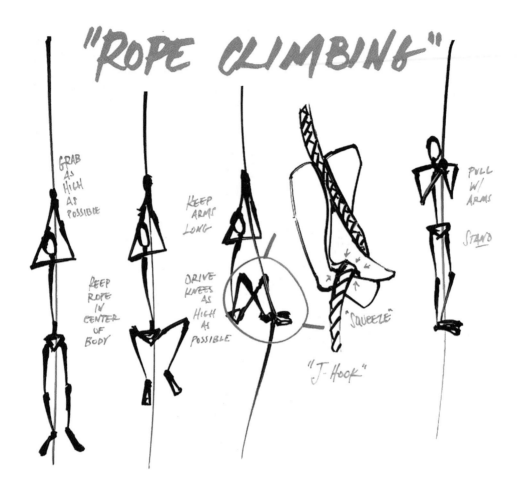

## Points of Performance

- Grip the rope.

- Move your knees as close as possible to your chest.

- Keep the rope in the center of your body.

- Wrap the rope on top of your dominant leg's foot.

- Step your free steps on the rope, pinching the rope between your feet.

- Pull with your arms while extending your hips and legs.

- Reach your arms overhead and release the wrapped rope to repeat the sequence.

# "WASH YOUR SHAKER BOTTLE AS SOON AS YOU'RE DONE."

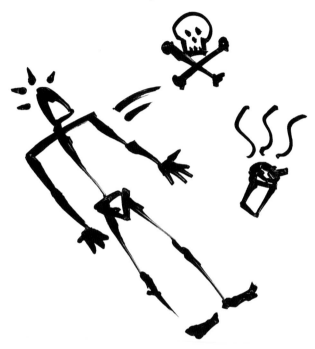

## What does this mean?

Wash (or at least rinse out) your shaker bottle as soon as you're finished using it, likely post-workout.

## Why is this important?

Failing to wash or rinse your shaker bottle (or remembering too late that you need to do it) will result in a stench that you will not soon forget. Worse still, bacteria will have taken up residence, and you'll have to sanitize your shaker bottle. I assure you, it only takes one time for you to understand the importance of this small task.

# CHAPTER ⑩

# PERSPECTIVE

# "BE A FOUNTAIN...

# ...NOT A DRAIN."

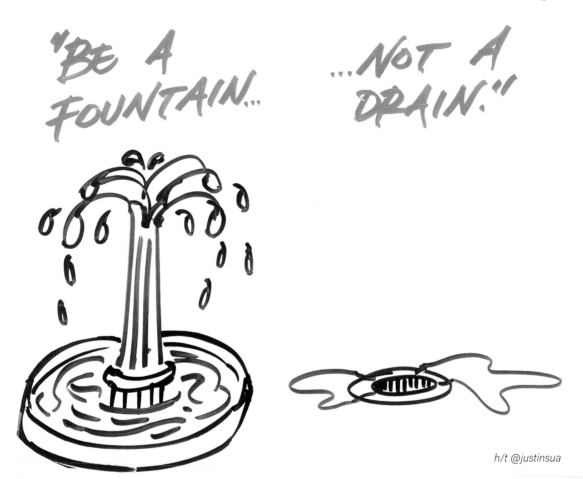

*h/t @justinsua*

## What does this mean?

Fountains bring life and energy to their team. They are positive and encouraging, and they make everyone around them better.

Drains suck the energy out of the room. They are negative, complain, and have a problem for every solution.

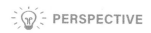 

# "A BIG SET IS JUST A LITTLE BAG OF CHIPS."

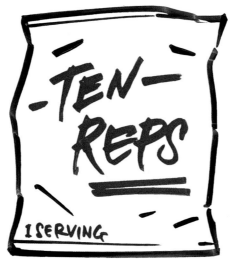

# "JUST EAT ONE CHIP AT A TIME!"

## What does this mean?

If you've ever eaten a bag of chips, at first you may think, "I won't eat this whole bag." Then you eat just one at a time. Before you know it, they're all gone!

## Why is this important?

You can use this perspective for any big task:

- A big set: Focus on one rep at a time
- A long row/run: Focus on one kilometer at a time

Don't focus on the whole bag, just eat one chip at a time!*

---

*This is NOT an encouragement to eat chips.

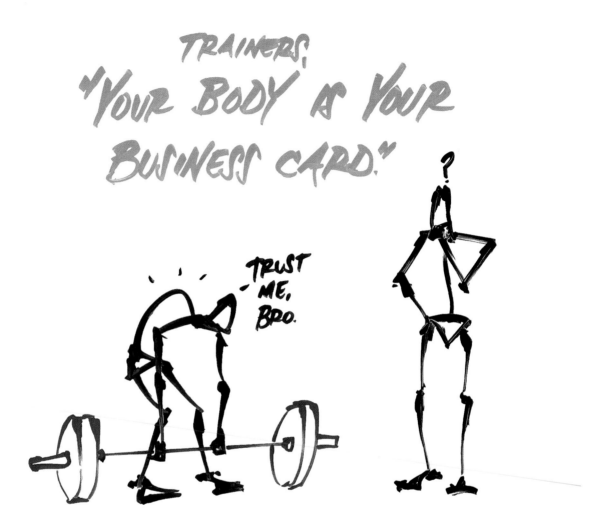

## What does this mean?

Looks aren't everything, but just like a business card, they do make a first impression.

How you move, present yourself, and act around others matters.

Don't look, move, or act like a trainer who appears to need a trainer.

Lead by example in all things. For example, if you set movement standards for your athletes, you should be displaying those same standards yourself. If you want to instill confidence within your athletes, display confidence yourself. Your body is a powerful tool. Be sure to use it properly.

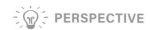 PERSPECTIVE

# "CALLUSES BUILD CHARACTER"

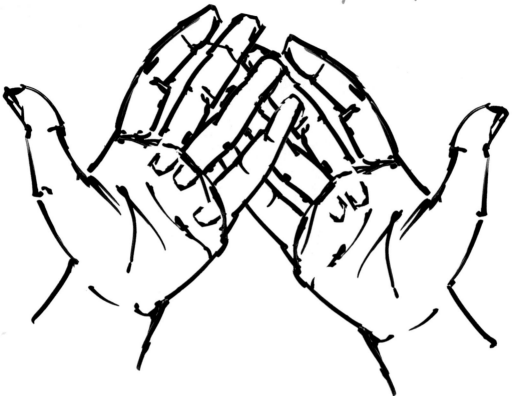

## What does this mean?

You learn a lot about yourself when you work hard.

When things get hard, when the weight gets heavy, when your grip starts to weaken, how do you react?

Do you stop?
Do you rest?
Do you press on?
How do you handle the stress?

It's no secret the lessons people learn during physical training directly apply to daily life. Get out there. Earn some calluses. Build some character. Learn more about who you are and who you can be.

*NOTE:* Take care of your hands. Shave or sand down your calluses. Don't let calluses get too big or they will rip. A ripped callus is similar to any other injury and can affect your training.

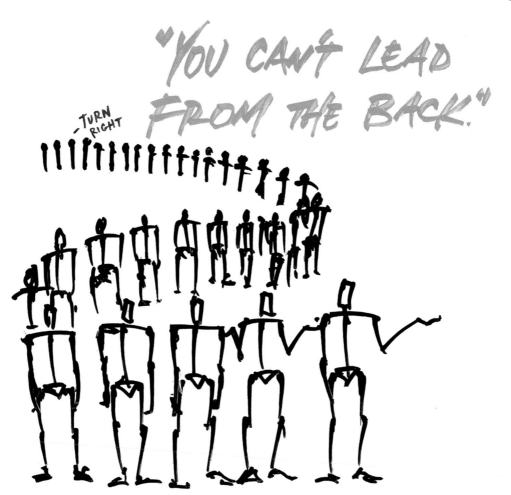

"YOU CAN'T LEAD FROM THE BACK."

- TURN RIGHT

## What does this mean?

Lead from the front. Use your voice *and* your actions.

Set the example.

Be the teammate you want to have on your team.

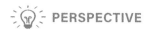 

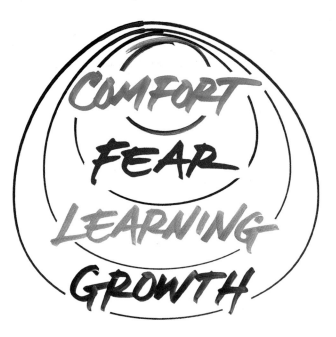

## What does this mean?

Although this graphic won't correspond to every situation for every person, growth is a lot like a multilayered gumball:

- **Comfort zone:** Feeling safe, unchallenged, in control
- **Fear zone:** Feeling uncertain, lacking confidence, making excuses
- **Learning zone:** Acquiring new skills to deal with challenges
- **Growth zone:** Achieving and setting new goals, developing confidence

## Why is this important?

It is necessary to gain the understanding that fear is often part of the growth process.

# CONSISTENCY & SUCCESS

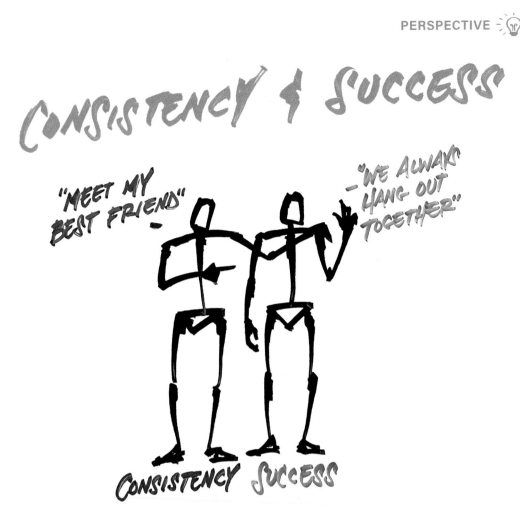

"MEET MY BEST FRIEND" -

- "WE ALWAYS HANG OUT TOGETHER"

CONSISTENCY    SUCCESS

## What does this mean?

Think of Consistency and Success as people. They are best friends who often hang out together. If you make friends with and start hanging out with Consistency, you will soon see his friend, Success. It takes consistency to find success.

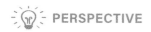
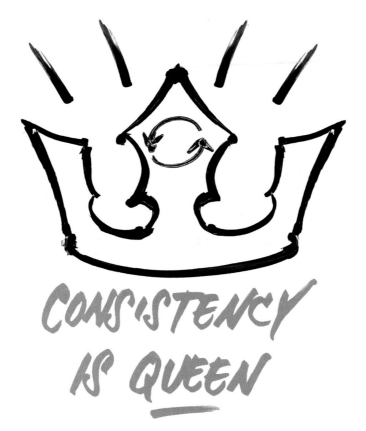

*h/t @olychad*

## What does this mean?

Strength, endurance, mobility, and skill are all earned over time. It is far more effective to consistently practice a little bit each day rather than randomly practice a whole bunch whenever you feel like it.

Consistency builds habits. Your habits are actions that lead to your success.

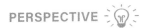

# "CONSISTENCY + WORK = PROGRESS"

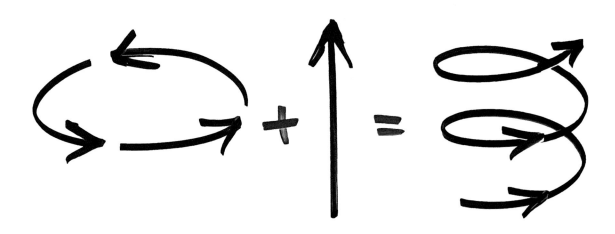

*h/t @eddiesmethod*

## What does this mean?

Consistency is vital to progress, but you need to be doing the *right things* consistently.

To make progress, the right things involve work. Add work to consistency, and you'll soon find progress.

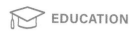 

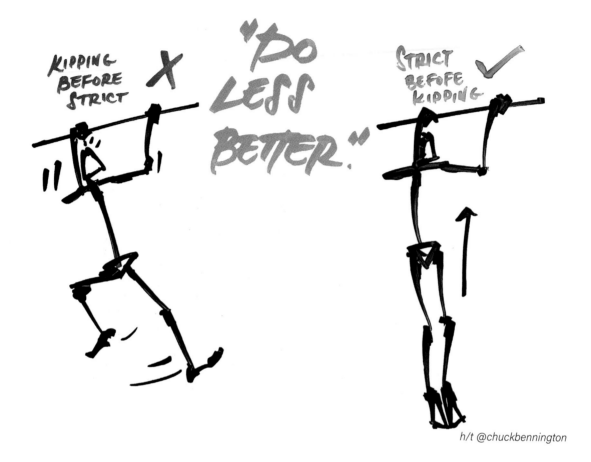

h/t @chuckbennington

## What does this mean?

Don't complicate things. Commit yourself to the basics.

## Why is this important?

To the beginner enthusiast, lighter weights and strict movements may not seem sexy. However, the technique gained through practicing the standards leads to proficiency and pushes the needle toward virtuosity—doing the common uncommonly well.

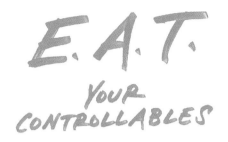

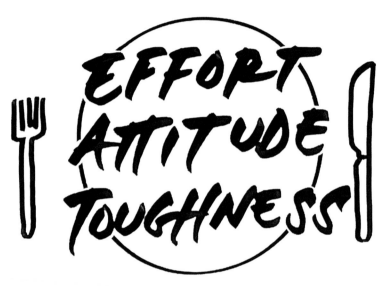

## What does this mean?

Focus on what you can control:

**E**ffort

**A**ttitude

**T**oughness

This common team philosophy applies to all areas of life as a recipe for success.

- **Effort:** Be the hardest worker in the room.

- **Attitude:** Be positive, humble, and enthusiastic.

- **Toughness:** Don't give up. If you get knocked down seven times, get back up eight.

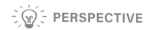

# "YOUR EGO IS NOT YOUR AMIGO"

*h/t @vndk8*

## What does this mean?

Ego is concerned about what others think.

Ego tells you to put more weight on the bar than you can handle.

Ego persuades you to scale UP a workout when you should be scaling it DOWN.

Ego leads to injury.

Ego is not your friend. Don't hang out with Ego.

## Why is this important?

Be humble and hungry. Be self-aware of your limitations but hungry in your desire to improve. Understanding that progress takes time and smaller steps leads to a longer journey.

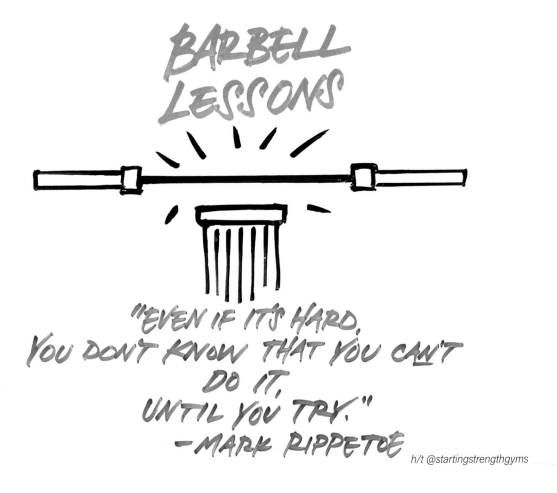

BARBELL LESSONS

"EVEN IF IT'S HARD,
YOU DON'T KNOW THAT YOU CAN'T
DO IT,
UNTIL YOU TRY."
—MARK RIPPETOE

*h/t @startingstrengthgyms*

## What does this mean?

If you allow yourself to give up on a rep or a certain amount of weight as soon as it gets challenging, you will never get stronger.

One of the greatest life lessons the barbell teaches you is that you don't know whether you can't do something unless you try it.

Before the set begins or before life challenges you, you must commit that you will try your hardest to overcome. Failing to do so limits your potential before the challenge even presents itself.

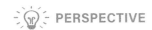 

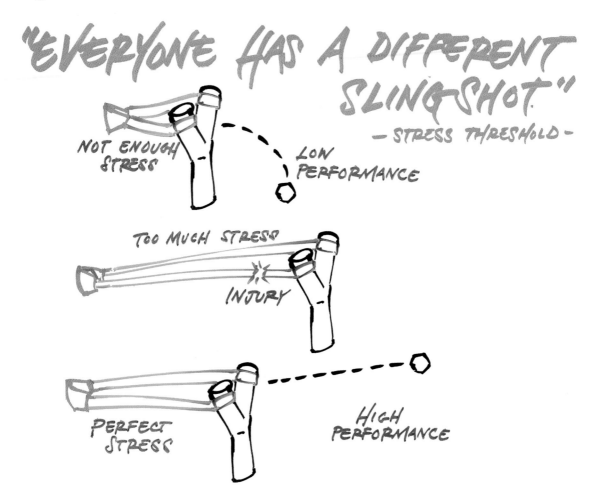

# "EVERYONE HAS A DIFFERENT SLINGSHOT."
## — STRESS THRESHOLD —

NOT ENOUGH STRESS

LOW PERFORMANCE

TOO MUCH STRESS

INJURY

PERFECT STRESS

HIGH PERFORMANCE

## What does this mean?

For a slingshot to work, stress must be applied; the leather pad must be pulled back to stretch the rubber.

In a similar fashion, an athlete improves when stress through training is applied. The amount of stress dictates the performance outcome:

- **Not enough stress:** Low performance
- **Too much stress:** Injury
- **Perfect stress:** High performance

## Why is this important?

Both the coach and athlete need to understand that each person has a different slingshot. Each athlete handles the stress of training differently. Therefore, the variables of training need to be personalized as well.

# "FITNESS MULTI-TOOL"
## YOUR FITNESS SKILL SET

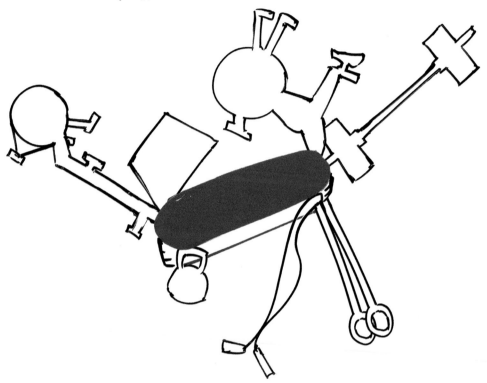

## What does this mean?

I picture the skills used to develop fitness ("fitness skill set") similar to a Swiss Army Knife or a Leatherman multi-tool. Each unique tool represents skills used to develop your fitness.

## Why is this important?

The more tools you develop, the more useful your fitness becomes, and the higher your general physical preparedness for everyday life will be.

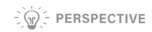
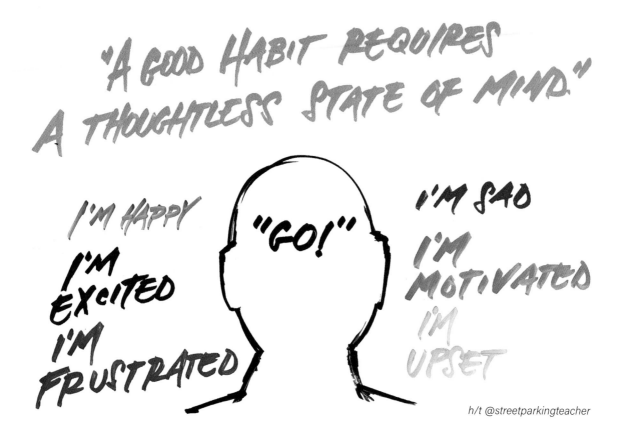

*"A GOOD HABIT REQUIRES A THOUGHTLESS STATE OF MIND."*

I'M HAPPY

I'M EXCITED

I'M FRUSTRATED

"GO!"

I'M SAD

I'M MOTIVATED

I'M UPSET

*h/t @streetparkingteacher*

**What does this mean?**

When you need to fulfill a healthy responsibility, don't overthink that decision—just do it. Overthinking leads to indecisiveness ("Maybe later would be better") or emotions ("I don't feel like doing this").

When it's time to do that thing you need to do, take on a thoughtless state of mind. Don't think; just go.

# "GRAY MATTER — MOVES → RED MATTER"

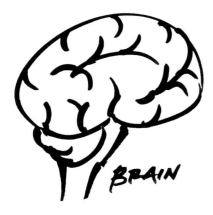

BRAIN

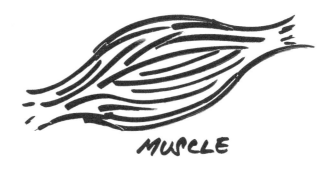

MUSCLE

## What does this mean?

Gray matter = your brain/mind

Red matter = your muscles

## Why is this important?

I often remind my students that we're not training only to strengthen our bodies in the weight room. We're also training to strengthen our minds, which is possibly of greater importance. The stronger your mind is, the stronger your body will become. It is the mind that drives the body. The gray matter moves the red matter.

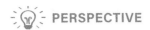
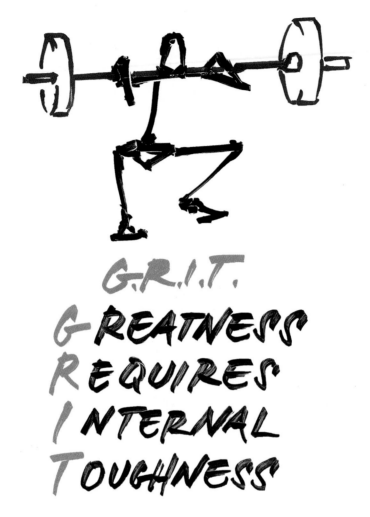

## What does this mean?

Grit means

- Pushing through when things are challenging
- Displaying courage during uncertainty
- Staying disciplined despite the absence of motivation

It all starts IN. YOUR. HEAD.

# HEAD DOWN, EYES FORWARD

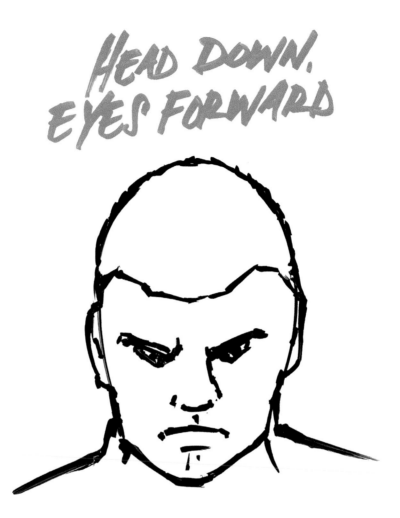

## What does this mean?

Mantras can be extremely valuable in sport performance. Like coaching cues, they help the athlete focus on what's important to methodically make progress.

I commonly use the mantra "head down, eyes forward" when it comes to training, especially in the middle of a hard session. Distractions tend to appear more powerful when you're fatigued. Mentally keeping your head down and eyes forward may help you or your athlete keep focused on the task at hand.

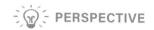
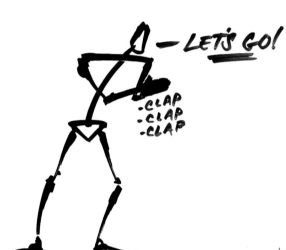

"IF YOUR PRESENCE DOESN'T MAKE AN IMPACT... YOUR ABSENCE WON'T MAKE A DIFFERENCE."

— LET'S GO!

·CLAP ·CLAP ·CLAP

*h/t @athletebydesign via @concord_strong/@skottiedoesntno*

## What does this mean?

Be a difference maker. In all of your relationships—as a coach, teammate, friend, or relative—create such a positive, valuable impact on others that you're missed when you're absent.

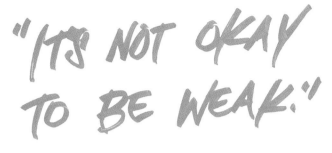

# "IT'S NOT OKAY TO BE WEAK."

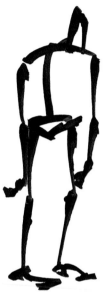

*h/t @jordan.b.peterson*

## What does this mean?

Weakness leads to and keeps you injured and sick.

Weakness lowers your quality of life and forces you to need assistance from others. Weakness keeps you from being the strongest version of yourself.

Weakness doesn't affect only you; it affects others around you as well. Be who you want to be, but be the strongest version of yourself.

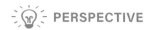
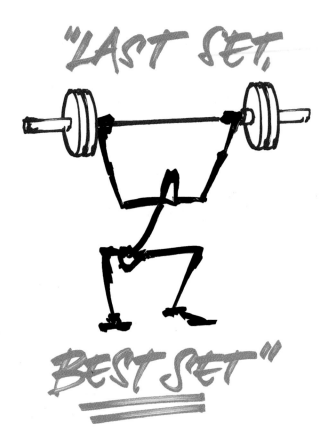

## What does this mean?

Finish strong!

By no means does this imply that earlier sets or intervals aren't important. However, the opportunities that lie within the push for the last set are extremely important and something you should look for each time you train.

If you have been pushing yourself, then you likely feel a little beat up and tired by the time you get to the last set. You may even feel a little scared or unsure of your capability (thinking, "Can I do this?").

Those last sets are the "golden moments" for you to capitalize on your gains: They

- Build physical strength

- Build mental toughness

- Build awareness of your limits

- Increase the importance of technique

# "PHYSICIANS ARE LIFEGUARDS. TRAINERS ARE SWIM COACHES."

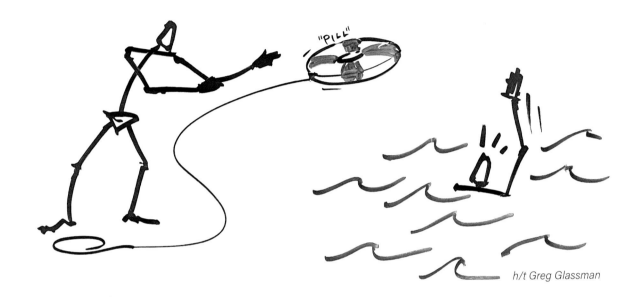

h/t Greg Glassman

## What does this mean?

If you have a good swim coach (a trainer), you are less likely to need a lifeguard (physician). Trainers and coaches are the front line for helping others live a healthy and fit life—a life that doesn't involve the need of a physician.

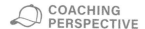

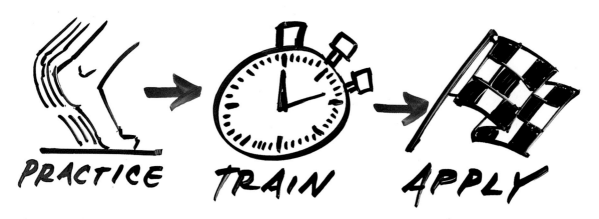

h/t @carlpaoli

**When?**

Creating progress

**What does this mean?**

The following steps create progress in whatever you want to do in life. For the purpose of this example, say you want to get better at playing basketball:

1. **Practice:** Take the time to deliberately work on a skill(s) relevant to your goal. Establish consistency and frequency for how often you do this (e.g., daily practice during basketball season).

2. **Train:** Similar to practice but now add a challenging element to the development of these skills. Test your progress, such as with a scrimmage against another team.

3. **Apply:** Take what you have developed in practice and strengthened in training and apply it to a specific moment. This would be like playing a basketball game against another team.

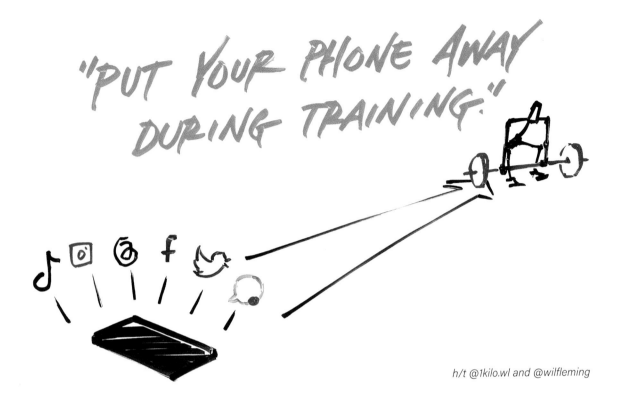

"PUT YOUR PHONE AWAY DURING TRAINING."

*h/t @1kilo.wl and @wilfleming*

## What does this mean?

Spend less time scrollin' and more time pullin'!

The best training comes from a focused mind. When you constantly allow yourself to become distracted by your phone, you simply will not reach your potential. Train with intent and purpose. Give your body the respect and attention it deserves during your training session. Save the scrolling on social media for later.

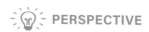
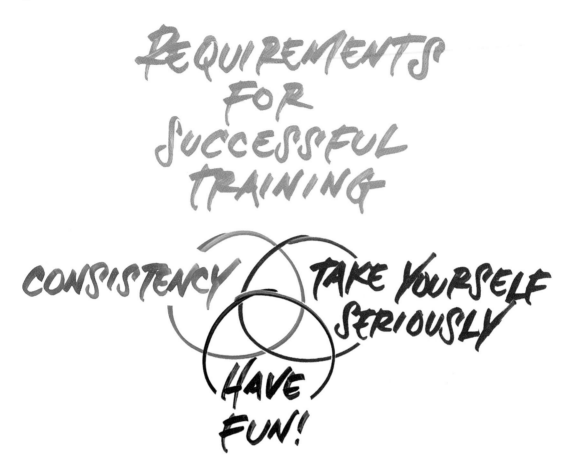

## What does this mean?

You're going to have a hard time being successful if you don't have these three things:

- **Consistency:** Getting stronger, building endurance, improving at a skill; these things don't just magically happen. It takes time, energy, and focus. To create progress, you must practice consistently.

- **Take yourself seriously:** Give yourself the respect you deserve. Set goals. Journal your progress. Get enough sleep. Eat the right foods. Set an intent and purpose for yourself.

- **Have fun!** If you don't find enjoyment, you'll dread your training and begin to avoid it. Do the type of training that you enjoy doing. Find others who enjoy the same training as well. Constantly learn from them. Celebrate your accomplishments.

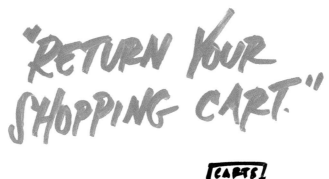

# "RETURN YOUR SHOPPING CART."

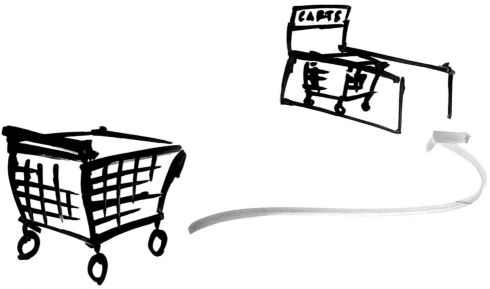

## What does this mean?

A responsible shopper returns a shopping cart to the cart corral when they're finished. Similarly, how you conduct yourself outside the gym reflects how you conduct yourself inside the gym.

Take ownership. Be responsible for your actions.

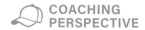

# WHEN YOU MAKE A MISTAKE:

# R.O.L.F. IT.

## Recognize it.
## Own it.
## Learn from it.
## Flush it.

*h/t @coachlisle*

## What does this mean?

Everyone makes mistakes, especially those people who are pushing themselves. When it happens to you (and it will), ROLF it:

- **Recognize it:** Understand what happened and what needs to change.

- **Own it:** Hold yourself accountable and don't blame others.

- **Learn from it:** Figure out why this happened and how to improve it.

- **Flush it:** Move on from it. Keep moving forward.

# ROUTINE NOT SUPERSTITION

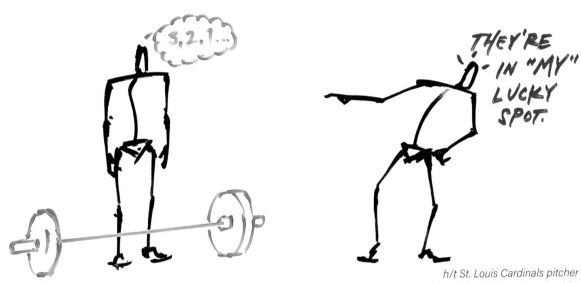

*h/t St. Louis Cardinals pitcher*
*Adam Wainwright via @redbirdriot*

## When?

Preparing to compete/perform (before a lift, race, etc.)

## What does this mean?

Establishing a personal routine before you do something provides a massive benefit. It prepares you both mentally and physically and provides a sense of familiarity to the setting.

However, know that circumstances beyond your control may keep you from following your exact routine. If you believe you must follow a precise sequence of steps to achieve success, you've created a superstition, which makes you a weaker competitor.

Establish a simple routine, not a superstition.

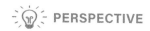
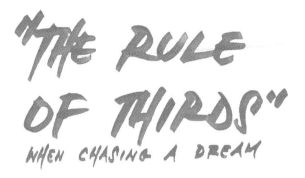

"THE RULE OF THIRDS"
WHEN CHASING A DREAM

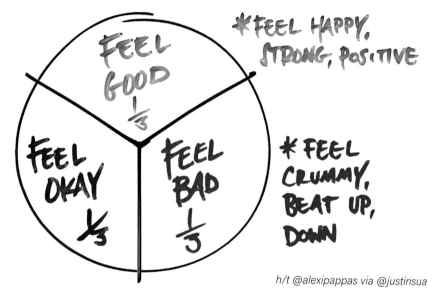

*FEEL HAPPY, STRONG, POSITIVE

FEEL GOOD 1/3

*FEEL ..OKAY

FEEL OKAY 1/3

FEEL BAD 1/3

* FEEL CRUMMY, BEAT UP, DOWN

*h/t @alexipappas via @justinsua*

## What does this mean?

When you're chasing a dream, do not be discouraged by bad days. You are meant to feel "good" one-third of the time, "bad" one-third of the time, and "okay" one-third of the time. If you are within these ratios, then you are doing fine!

If you are feeling good more than a third of the time, you may not be pushing hard enough.

If you are feeling bad more than a third of the time, you may be pushing yourself too much.

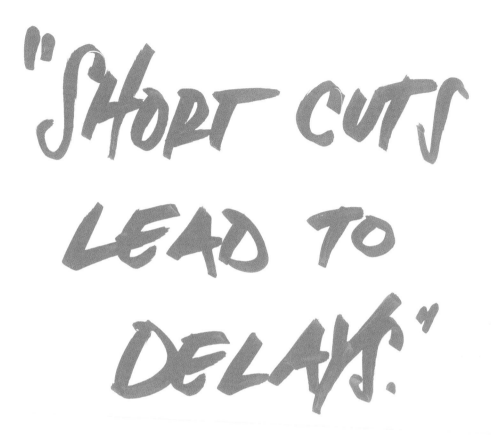

"SHORT CUTS LEAD TO DELAYS."

## What does this mean?

The solution to most problems is consistent hard work.

However, generally speaking, people want to see quick results and will typically do whatever it takes to avoid consistent hard work.

Over time, short cuts fail, and people who try them end up spending more time working toward their goal. If they'd stayed with the original plan and put in consistent hard work, they'd reach the goal quicker.

Do it the right way the first time.

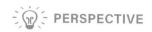 

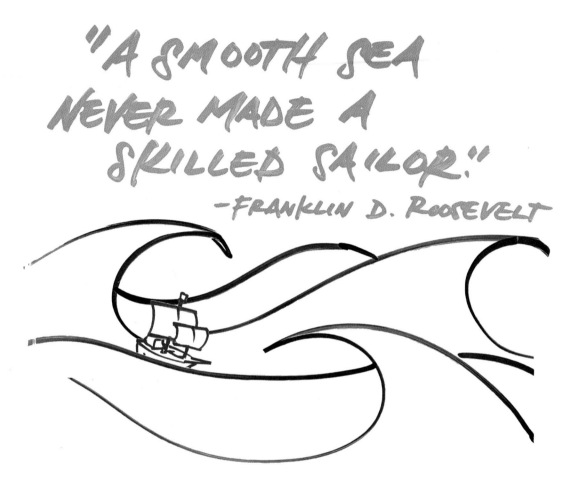

"A SMOOTH SEA NEVER MADE A SKILLED SAILOR."

—FRANKLIN D. ROOSEVELT

### What does this mean?

This quote from Franklin D. Roosevelt means life will inevitably bring you (the sailor) challenges and conflict (stormy seas). When these things happen, do not let yourself become frustrated or dismayed. Instead, use these circumstances to strengthen your skills.

Growth, progress, and strength don't happen without overcoming adversity.

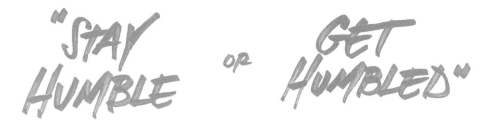

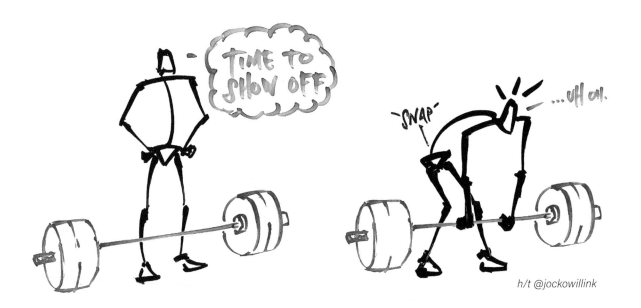

h/t @jockowillink

## What does this mean?

As a coach, you are a teacher. Good teachers are forever students—constantly learning from others.

The more you learn from others, the more you realize how much more there is to learn.

You must have the humility to understand that you may know a lot, but you will never know everything.

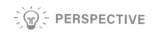 

# 🔍 | "SUBSTITUTE FOR HARD WORK"

## NO RESULTS FOR:
### "SUBSTITUTE FOR HARD WORK"

## DID YOU MEAN:
### "HOW TO MAKE EXCUSES"

**What does this mean?**

You can search Google for a "fitness hack." You can get inspired by a fitness influencer. You can buy the latest fitness gear. You can even Photoshop your selfie photos.

You can search for ways around doing hard work, but they are all just excuses.

Goals worth achieving are accomplished with hard work. Period. Work wins.

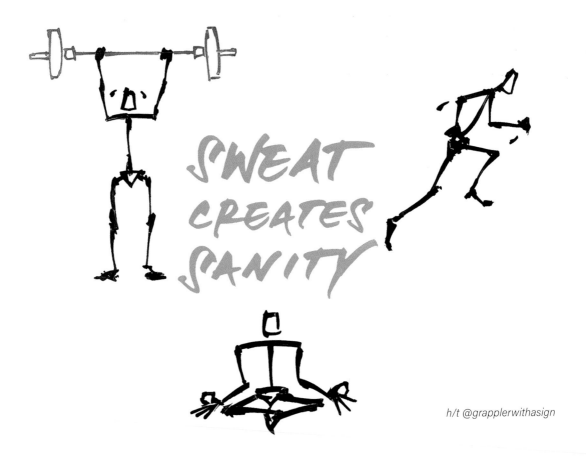

SWEAT CREATES SANITY

*h/t @grapplerwithasign*

## What does this mean?

Simply put, regular physical exercise benefits both your body and your mind.

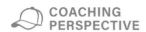
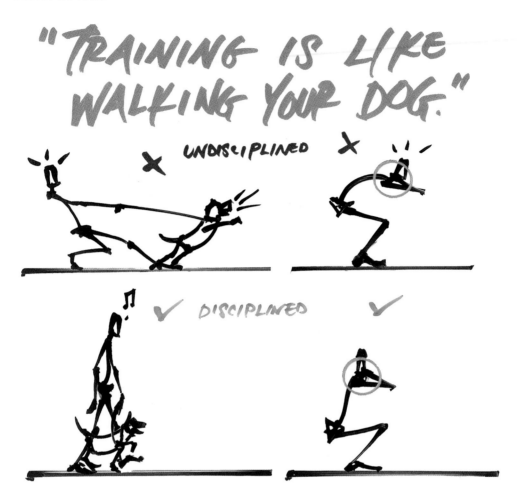

## What does this mean?

When I walk my dog but ignore him, he pulls me all over the place and barks at other dogs. My lack of discipline teaches him bad habits. However, if I pay attention to him and consistently and immediately react when he pulls or barks, he learns how to behave correctly. In both instances, I'm walking my dog. However, one method improves his performance, whereas the other worsens it.

The same goes for training. If you never practice good mechanics, you teach yourself bad habits that eventually lead to stalled progress or injury. However, if you consistently pay attention to your positioning, you move more efficiently.

In both instances, you're training. However, one method improves your performance and keeps you safer.

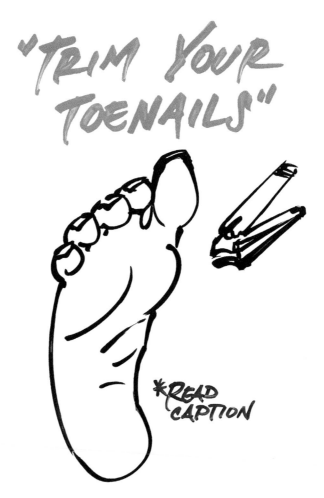

# "TRIM YOUR TOENAILS"

*READ CAPTION

## What does this mean?

Take time to take care of yourself. Do simple things:

- Drink enough water.
- Spend time mobilizing your body.
- Read a chapter in a book.
- Trim your toenails.

## Why is this important?

When you are overwhelmed (or being lazy), it can be easy to allow yourself to be distracted from the simple things that can improve your self-care. (Plus, you really should take better care of your feet.)

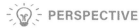
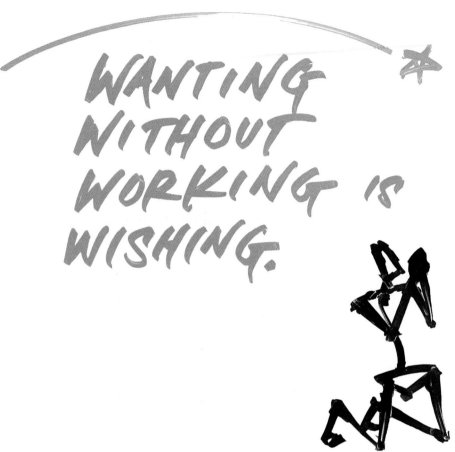

## WANTING WITHOUT WORKING IS WISHING.

### What does this mean?

If you want anything good, you must put in the work. Period.

You can't wish or hope for it to happen.

Work wins.

# WARM-UP = PREHEATING

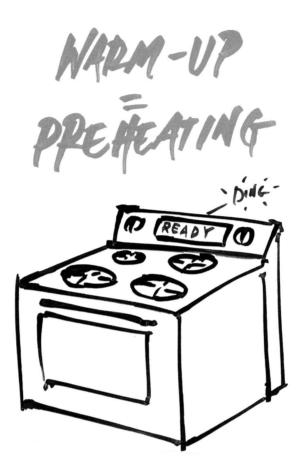

h/t @bamfhammer

## What does this mean?

Treat your warm-up like you are preheating your oven.

When baking something to eat, you get the best results when you preheat the oven to the prescribed temperature before you put in the food. This takes planning, patience, and attention to detail.

In the same respect, get the most out of your training by properly warming up beforehand.

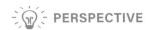
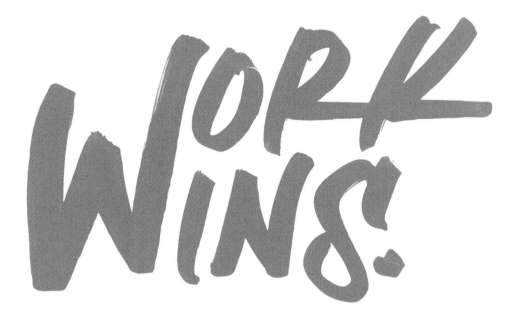

## What does this mean?

Wins of significance, such as personal bests, accomplishing goals, and maintaining consistency, don't happen passively.

These things take dedicated effort. If you want to make progress in the things that you care about, it takes work. Period.

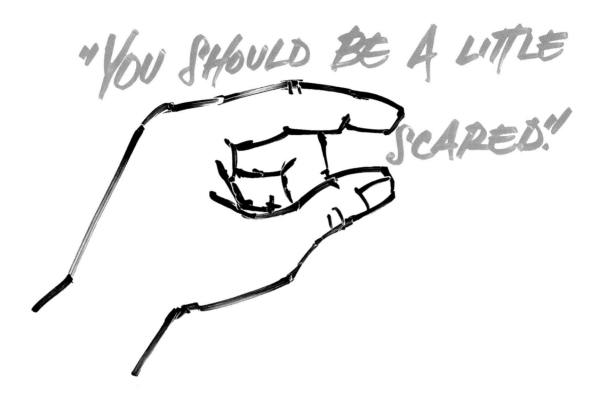

"YOU SHOULD BE A LITTLE SCARED."

## What does this mean?

Before your training session, you should be a little scared. Some element of the session should make you feel at least a little fear—something that makes you second-guess your ability.

## Why is this important?

A little fear is a good thing.

It is through fear that you deal with uncertainty and discomfort; in turn, you acquire new skills, develop confidence, and build strength.

It is within the fear that you step up to the challenge. Accepting the challenge helps you become a stronger version of yourself.

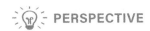 

# "YOUR BLAME IS YOUR CHAIN."

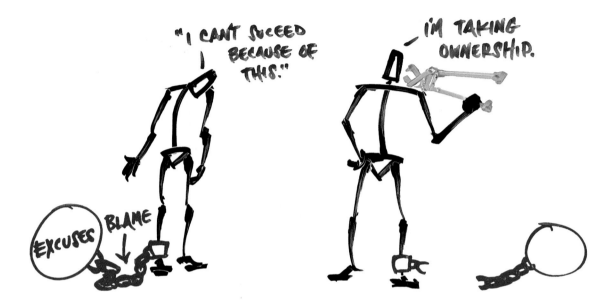

## What does this mean?

When you blame others for things that go wrong in your life, you become a slave to those excuses.

- "It's *their* fault I'm in this position."
- "It's because of *them* that I'm in this situation."
- "We're losing because of *them*."

You're placing the outcome of your success on someone or something else. Your *blame* chains you to your excuse.

Break the chain! Take ownership of your situation and do something about it. There is such great freedom in realizing that it's up to *you* to do something about it.

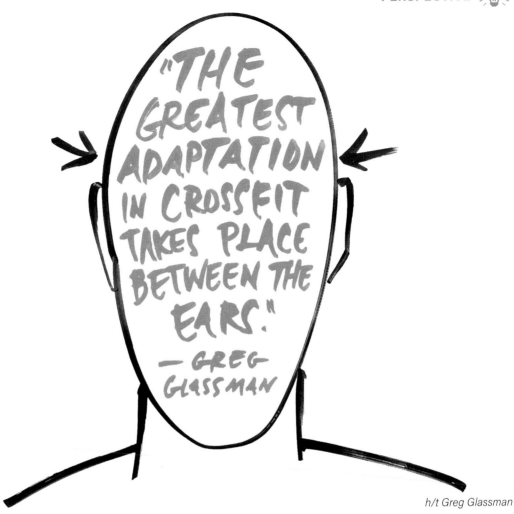

*h/t Greg Glassman*

## What does this mean?

As with other sports, physical training is a catalyst for the psychological development and growth of the individual.

## Why is this important?

The mind moves the body. Strengthen the mind to strengthen the body.

For more information please see "Coaching the Mental Side of CrossFit" by Greg Amundson 2010 in the @crossfittraining Journal.

# CHAPTER (11)

## POSITIONING

# "BICEP BY THE EAR"
## SINGLE ARM OHS

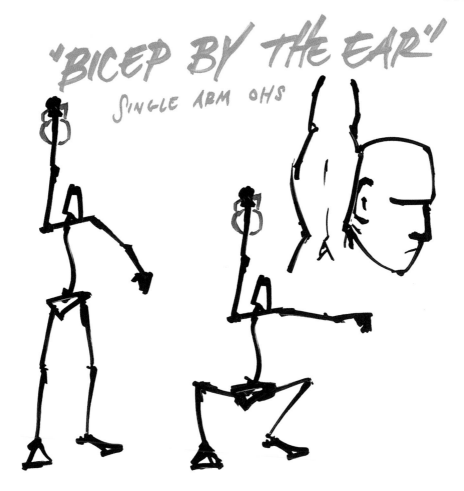

## When?

Single arm overhead squatting

## What does this mean?

When holding an object overhead with a single arm (kettlebell, dumbbell, medicine ball, etc.), you want to keep it as close to your midline as possible and have a locked-out elbow.

Keeping the biceps of the supporting arm next to the ear keeps the weight of that object close to your midline.

## Why is this important?

Keeping the object close to your midline places you in a balanced, efficient, stable position.

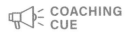
# "BONES DON'T GET TIRED"
## — STACKED POSITIONING —

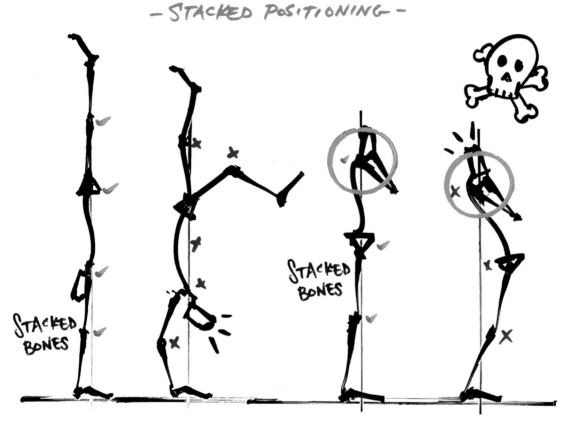

STACKED
BONES

STACKED
BONES

### When?
This crossover cue can be used to describe positioning in gymnastics and Olympic lifting.

### What does this mean?
A stacked position (joints locked out and bones stacked on top of each other) is more efficient than a slouched position.

### Why is this important?
In a stacked position, you use less energy and move more efficiently.

# "KEEP IT TIGHT TO KEEP IT LIGHT"

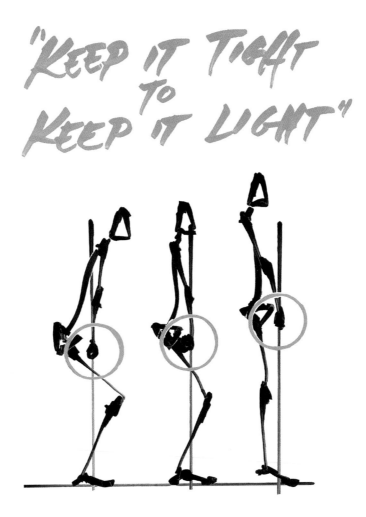

## When?

Picking weight up off the ground

## What does this mean?

When moving weight on a barbell, keep it tight to the body to keep the bar feeling as light as possible.

## Why is this important?

Keeping the barbell close to your body is a more efficient use of power than letting it move away from you. The farther the weight is from your body, the heavier it'll feel.

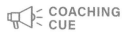
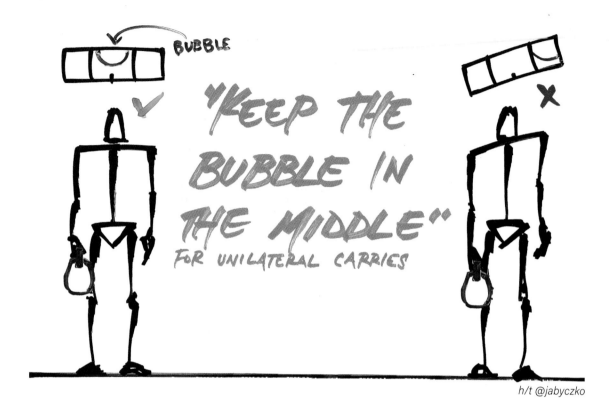

h/t @jabyczko

## When?

Unilateral carries

## What does this mean?

Imagine a level used for construction is resting on your shoulders during a unilateral carry. Keep your shoulders level so the bubble stays in the middle.

## Why is this important?

Unilateral carries are movements where one side of the body (right or left) is carrying more than the other. These movements are used in training for multiple reasons. They increase proprioception, or your body's awareness of positioning and movement. This type of training also addresses imbalances within your body. For example, your right side may be stronger than your left side. Additionally, unilateral carries can help with stability throughout a range of movement.

The value in unilateral carries comes from fighting against the resistance on one side to maintain your balance and posture—"keeping the bubble in the middle." Letting that bubble drift to one side is letting the weight win.

# "KEEP POWER IN THE BUCKET"

### DESCRIBING A POWER LEAK

#### E.G. FIRST PULL

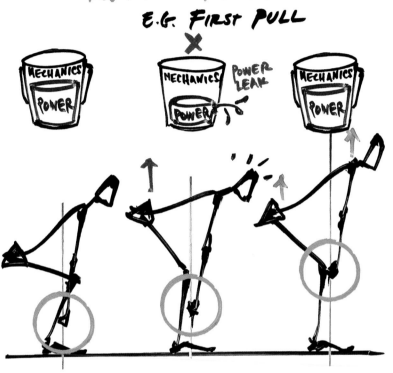

## When?

Describing a power leak

## What does this mean?

Mechanics are the bucket. Power is the water. Movement inefficiencies are leaks.

Simply put, a power leak is wasted energy.

For example, a common power leak of the first pull is the hips rising faster than the shoulders.

Here are some cues to address this power leak:

- Hips and shoulders rise together.
- Chest first.
- Avoid the "stripper booty."

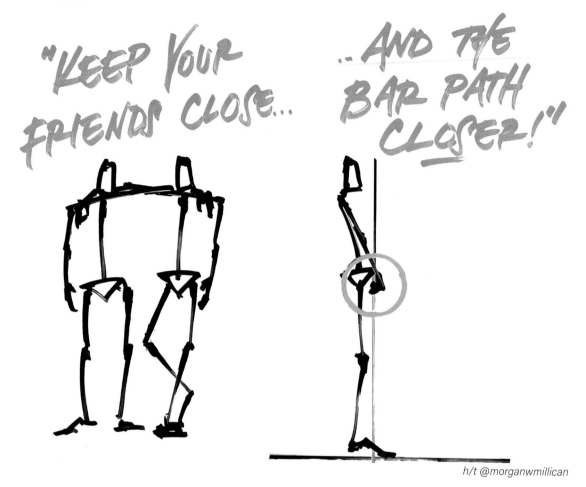

*"KEEP YOUR FRIENDS CLOSE...*

*..AND THE BAR PATH CLOSER!"*

*h/t @morganwmillican*

### When?

Clean and snatch

### What does this mean?

Just like you keep close contact with your friends, keep the bar path close to your body.

### Why is this important?

The most important factor to being consistent and efficient in the snatch and clean is to keep the bar as close to your center of gravity as possible and the velocity of the path as smooth as possible.

# "LIKE A WHIP"

### DESCRIBING CORE TO EXTREMITY MOVEMENT
### E.G. PUSH PRESS

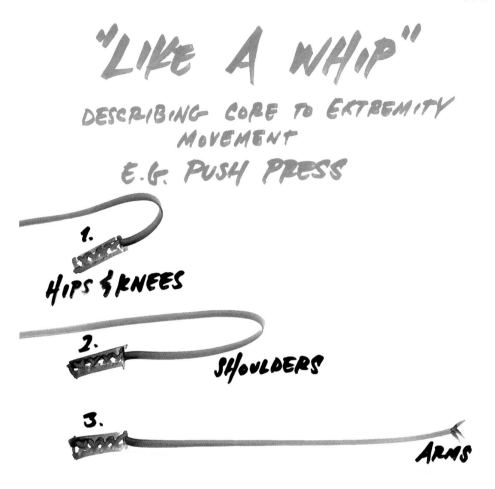

1. HIPS & KNEES

2. SHOULDERS

3. ARMS

## When?

Describing core to extremity movement

## What does this mean?

Functional movement begins at the core of the body and radiates toward the extremities.

In the push press example shown

1. Your trunk establishes midline stability. Your hips dip down, your knees bend, and both drive to extension.

2. Power travels outward to your legs and shoulders.

3. Power launches the bar off the front rack, and your shoulders and arms push through to finish.

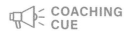
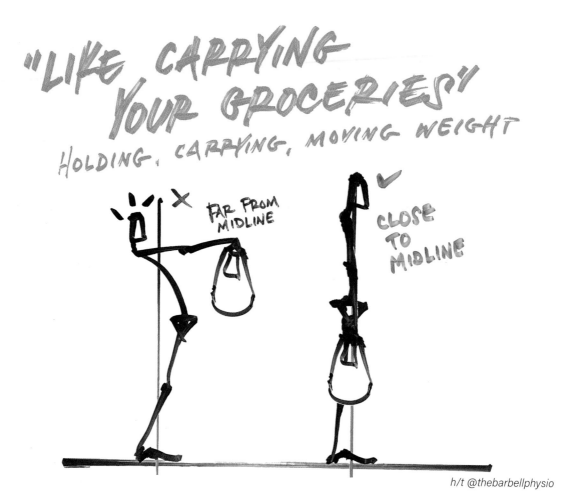

"LIKE CARRYING YOUR GROCERIES"

HOLDING, CARRYING, MOVING WEIGHT

X FAR FROM MIDLINE

✔ CLOSE TO MIDLINE

*h/t @thebarbellphysio*

## When?

Efficiently holding, carrying, and moving weight

## What does this mean?

Regardless of whether you're carrying a barbell or a bag of groceries, the laws of physics are the same. The closer the object is to your center of gravity, the more efficient the movement will be. Next time you're carrying groceries, pay attention to your positioning. You are likely demonstrating functional movement without even knowing it!

# "LIKE PUSHING A DOOR OPEN"
## DEADLIFT, SQUAT, CLEAN, SNATCH

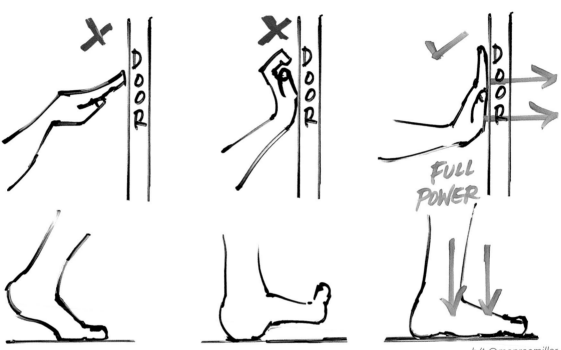

FULL POWER

*h/t @monroemiller*

## When?

Deadlift, squatting variations, cleans, snatches, etc.

## What does this mean?

When you push a door open, you use your whole hand rather than your fingertips or the heel. Similarly, whenever you're pushing your feet into the ground, push with your full foot.

## Why is this important?

Pushing with your full foot transfers as much power as possible *and* helps keep your system balanced throughout the movement.

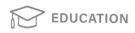
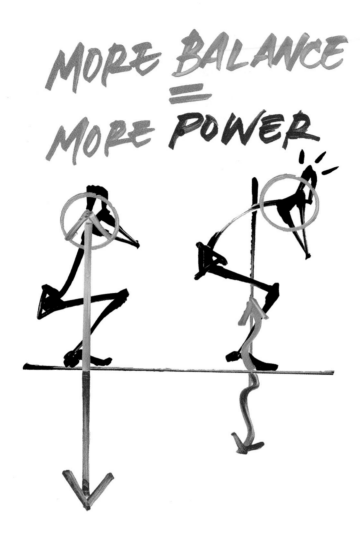

## When?

All functional movement

## What does this mean?

The more balanced you are under or over the bar, the more power you can push into the ground.

## How do you improve balance?

- Increase mobility
- Slow down your lifts
- Drill positions through variations
- Stop wearing overengineered footwear

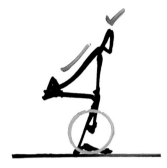

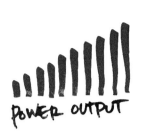

POWER OUTPUT

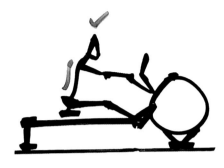

"POSITION DETERMINES POWER"

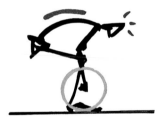

POWER OUTPUT

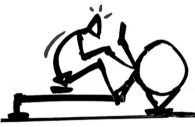

## When?

All functional movement

## What does this mean?

The weaker your position, the lower your power output potential. The stronger your position, the greater your power output potential.

Practice your positioning!

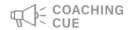

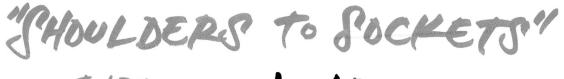

## "SHOULDERS TO SOCKETS"

— TO ACTIVATE LATS, TRAPS, & DELTS —

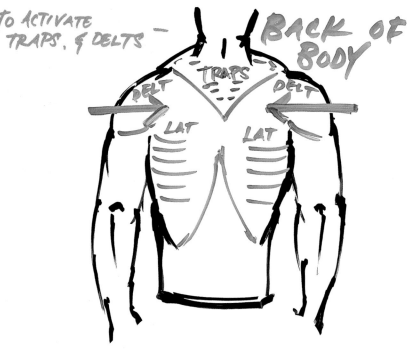

### When?

Engaging the lats, delts, and traps

### What does this mean?

Pull your shoulders into their sockets. By doing so, you activate the musculature that allows you to stabilize your upper body.

This engagement is commonly seen in many athletic positions, including

- Deadlifts
- Kettlebell cleans
- Ring support position
- Jumping rope
- Even engaging the lats during bench press

Additionally, a common miscue is "shoulders back," which does not target engaging the strong lats and can lead to hyperextension of the torso.

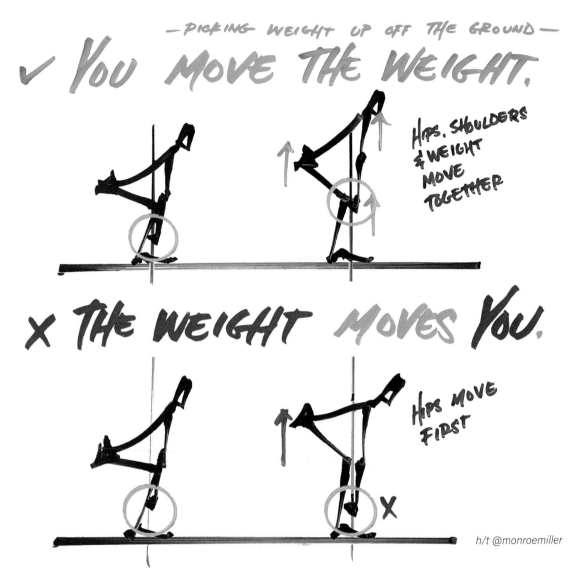

— PICKING WEIGHT UP OFF THE GROUND —

✓ You MOVE THE WEIGHT.

HIPS. SHOULDERS & WEIGHT MOVE TOGETHER

✗ THE WEIGHT MOVES You.

HIPS MOVE FIRST

h/t @monroemiller

## When?

Picking weight up off the ground

## What does this mean?

Prior to lifting, take a breath, brace, and then move the weight with your body. Your hips and shoulders and the weight should all move at the same time.

## Why is this important?

Upon initiation of lifting the weight (barbell, dumbbell, kettlebell) off the ground, if any body part moves before the actual weight moves, your body is leaking power, which is probably placing you in a less efficient position.

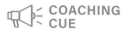
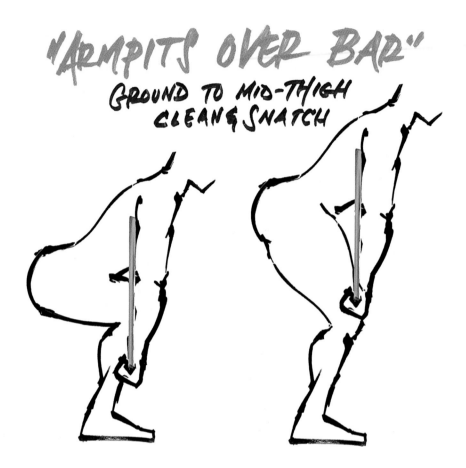

"ARMPITS OVER BAR"
GROUND TO MID-THIGH
CLEAN & SNATCH

### When?

Body/bar position from ground to mid-thigh of clean and snatch

### What does this mean?

Keep your armpits over the bar throughout the first pull (from the ground to mid-thigh).

### Why is this important?

Maintaining alignment with your armpits over the bar helps place you in the optimal balanced position for entry into the second pull of the lift—the final upward explosion.

# "HINGE LIKE BARBIE"
## —HIP HINGE MOVEMENTS—

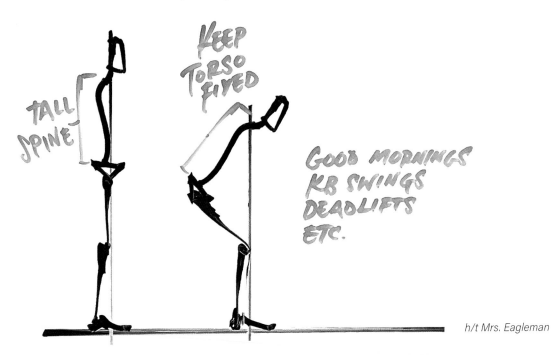

TALL SPINE

KEEP TORSO FIXED

GOOD MORNINGS
KB SWINGS
DEADLIFTS
ETC.

*h/t Mrs. Eagleman*

## When?

Hinge movements, such as good mornings, kettlebell swings, and deadlifts

## What does this mean?

When a doll bends at the hip, the torso stays in a fixed position. In a similar fashion, throughout the hip hinge movement, as you move your hips back, you should hold your spine in a neutral position.

## Why is this important?

The ability to properly load the hips enables you to generate the most power during extension.

# CHAPTER (12)

## BENCH PRESS

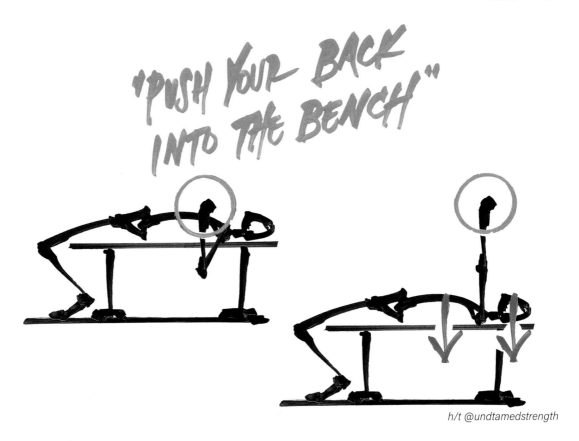

*"PUSH YOUR BACK INTO THE BENCH"*

*h/t @undtamedstrength*

### When?

Bench press

### What does this mean?

When setting your arch during the setup and rep(s) of the bench press, adjust your positioning so you're pushing as much of your upper back into the bench as possible. Do this by arching your lower back and pulling your shoulder blades together. Push your feet into the ground through a leg drive to create stability on the bench throughout your entire lower body.

### Why is this important?

Proper engagement throughout your entire body creates a stable base for the chest and arms to move the bar.

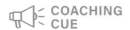
# "BOOTIE ON BENCH"
## — BENCH PRESS —

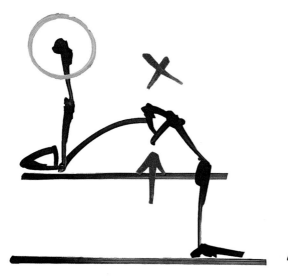

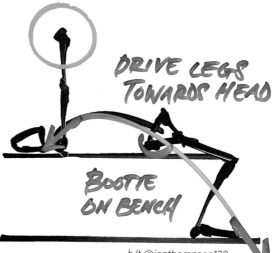

DRIVE LEGS TOWARDS HEAD

BOOTIE ON BENCH

*h/t @jenthompson132*

## When?

Bench press

## What does this mean?

During the setup and throughout the rep(s) of the bench press, keep your rear end touching the bench.

## Why is this important?

A lifter performing a well-executed bench press employs their lower body and core to create a stable base of support. They do this by setting the arch of the torso and driving their legs into the ground.

A common error with beginner lifters during the leg drive is pushing their hips skyward rather than back toward the shoulders, which creates a loss of power.

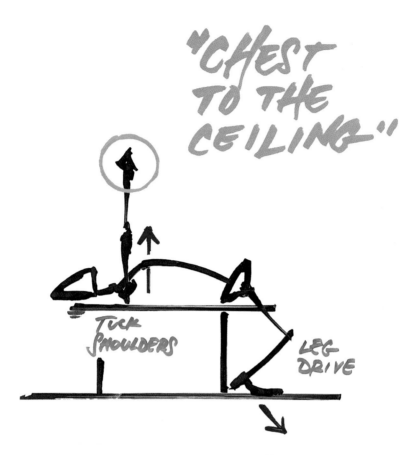

"CHEST TO THE CEILING"

TUCK SHOULDERS

LEG DRIVE

*h/t @untamedstrength*

## When?

Bench press

## What does this mean?

During the setup and throughout each rep of the bench press, drive your chest to the ceiling by packing your shoulder blades together and under your back. Additionally, position your feet so you can apply pressure to the ground without your hips leaving the bench.

## Why is this important?

Driving your chest to the ceiling:

- Shortens the range of motion for the bar path
- Engages the muscles in your upper back

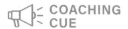
# "EYEBROWS UNDER THE BAR"
## BENCH PRESS SETUP

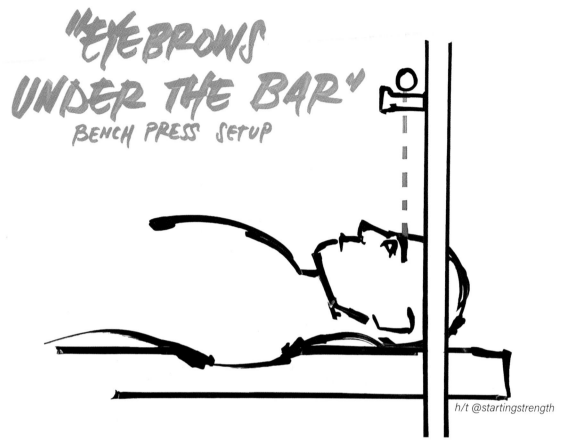

h/t @startingstrength

## When?

Setting up for bench press

## What does this mean?

A common error demonstrated by new lifters is setting up for the bench press with their bodies positioned too far back on the bench. Consequently, the J-cups are directly in the path of the bar during extension.

To remedy this, lie down with your eyes looking straight up. Adjust yourself on the bench so your eyebrows are directly underneath the barbell when it is on the rack.

## Why is this important?

This position keeps you close enough to the uprights to unrack the bar safely and efficiently but far enough away so that you don't hit the J-cups when pressing the bar back up.

For more information, check out "Learning to Bench Press | The Starting Strength Method" on YouTube.

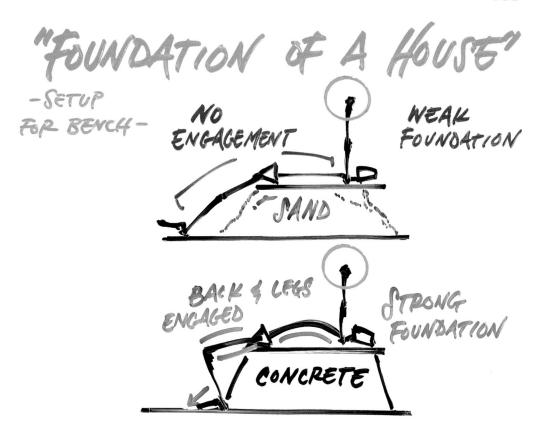

# "FOUNDATION OF A HOUSE"

-SETUP FOR BENCH-

NO ENGAGEMENT

WEAK FOUNDATION

SAND

BACK & LEGS ENGAGED

STRONG FOUNDATION

CONCRETE

## When?

Setup for bench press

## What does this mean?

Similar to the way the foundation of a house determines its strength, your setup during the bench press determines your potential for lifting weight.

Weak foundation (sand) = no engagement from back and lower body

Strong foundation (concrete) = "set your arch":

- Lift your chest as high as possible.
- Drive your upper traps into the bench.
- Retract and depress your shoulder blades.
- Keep your glutes flexed.
- Push aggressively into the floor.

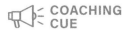

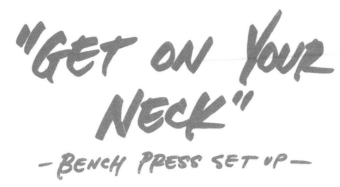

"GET ON YOUR NECK"

—BENCH PRESS SET UP—

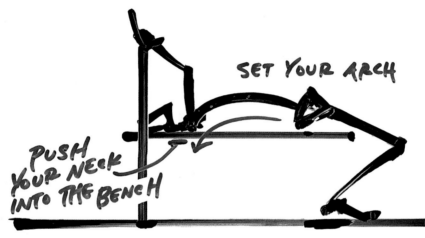

SET YOUR ARCH

PUSH YOUR NECK INTO THE BENCH

*h/t @jplifts423*

## When?

Bench press

## What does this mean?

During your setup for the bench press, pull your shoulder blades back and down and press as much of your neck flat into the bench as possible.

## Why is this important?

This small detail helps create a stronger arched position through the thoracic spine while anchoring your body to the bench. This position establishes a strong connection for your body to move the barbell.

# "KNUCKLES UP"
## FOR BENCH PRESS

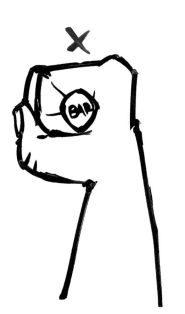 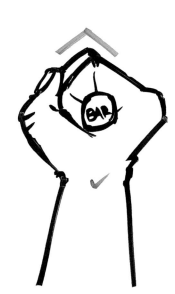 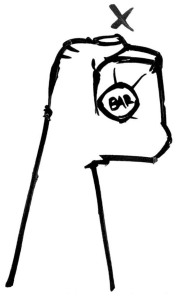

*h/t @untamedstrength*

## When?
Bench press

## What does this mean?
Your first, middle, and last knuckle should make an arrow and point straight to the ceiling during the bench press.

## Why is this important?
Pointing your knuckles to the ceiling creates a more stable connection with the bar and a more efficient power transfer through your arms by keeping it stacked over your wrist.

# CHAPTER (13)

## ROWING

# "BREAK THE GLASS WALL"

### – THE DRIVE DURING ROWING –

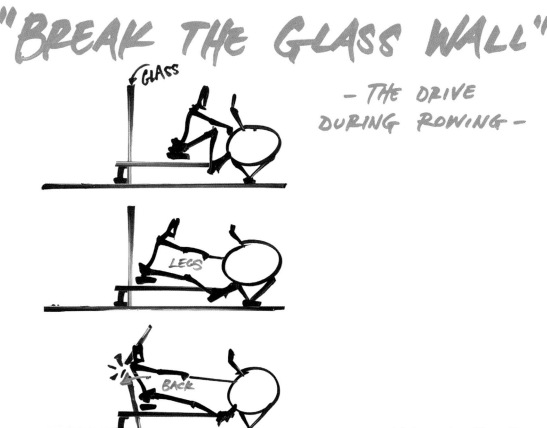

GLASS

LEGS

BACK

THEN ARMS

*h/t @gracechapcf Grace Chapman*

## When?

Rowing

## What does this mean?

The hips and legs are massive power generators, especially during rowing. A common error is when the rower rushes to finish the stroke and uses their arms prior to extending their hips (or without extending them at all).

Imagine there is a glass wall behind you when you're rowing. Make sure you extend your legs before your hips and then break the glass wall before you bend your arms.

## Why is this important?

This technique improves your movement efficiency and increases your power output.

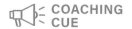
# "THINK DEADLIFT, NOT SQUAT"

## — ROWING: CATCH POSITION —

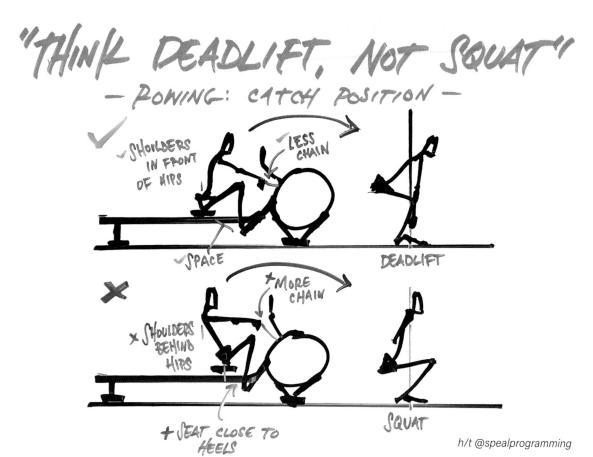

✓ SHOULDERS IN FRONT OF HIPS

LESS CHAIN

✓ SPACE

DEADLIFT

✗ SHOULDERS BEHIND HIPS

+ MORE CHAIN

+ SEAT CLOSE TO HEELS

SQUAT

*h/t @spealprogramming*

### When?

Rowing

### What does this mean?

During the catch and drive of the rowing stroke, your hips and shoulders should move together as your legs drive. This is similar to the mechanics of the deadlift. Your shoulders should start slightly in front of your hips at the catch and remain slightly in front of your hips as your legs drive until the legs are almost fully extended.

### Why is this important?

This technique prevents you from losing distance on the chain, and it gives you the opportunity for more leg drive.

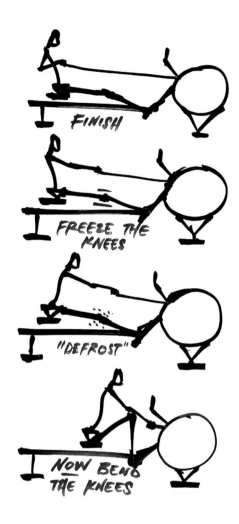

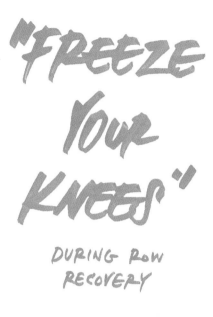

"FREEZE YOUR KNEES"

DURING ROW RECOVERY

*h/t @alicia_r_clark via @ucanrow2*

## When?

During the rowing stroke recovery

## What does this mean?

A common mistake people make during the recovery of the rowing stroke is to immediately bend their knees after the finish. Instead, "freeze" your knees, allow your arms to extend and then rock your shoulders forward.

Think of the handle "defrosting" your knees as it passes them. After your knees are "defrosted," bend your knees and roll forward to the catch position.

## Why is this important?

This technique sets your body in a stronger position for the catch and maximizes the efficiency of your leg drive.

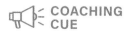
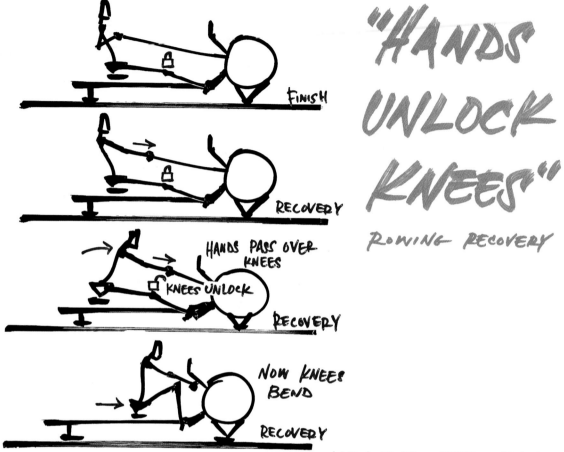

"HANDS UNLOCK KNEES"

ROWING RECOVERY

h/t @sdm_7.7 of @crossfit617/@crossfit617braintree

### When?

Rowing recovery

### What does this mean?

During the recovery,

- Extend your arms until they straighten before you lean from your hips toward the flywheel.

- Once your hands have cleared your knees, allow your knees to bend ("hands unlock knees") and gradually slide the seat forward on the monorail.

- For your next stroke, return to the catch position with your shoulders relaxed and your shins vertical.

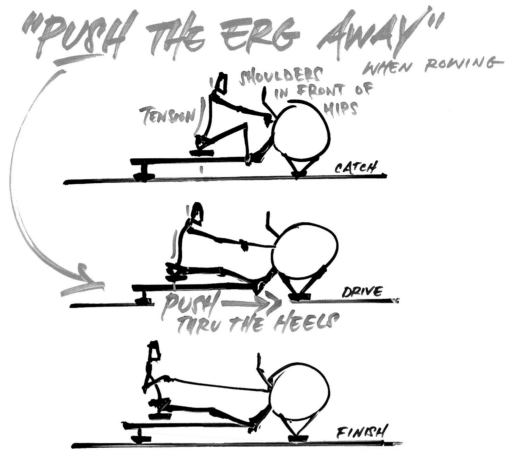

# "PUSH THE ERG AWAY"

WHEN ROWING

SHOULDERS IN FRONT OF HIPS

TENSION

CATCH

PUSH → THRU THE HEELS

DRIVE

FINISH

*h/t @cfkate*

## When?

Rowing

## What does this mean?

Rowing is a pushing sport, not a pulling sport. During the initial drive of the stroke, think of pushing the erg away from your body with your legs. Starting the stroke with this leg drive is crucial to leading to an efficient movement pattern: legs, back, and then arms.

## Why is this important?

This sequence enables you to maximize the force production of your entire body rather than using only your back and arms.

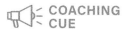
# "ROCK BEFORE YOU ROLL"

### DURING ROWING STROKE RECOVERY

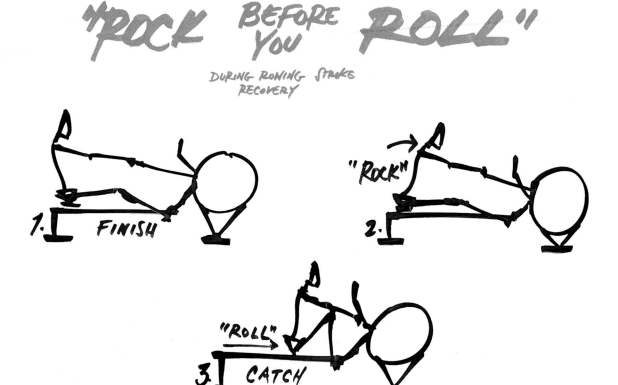

1. FINISH

2. "ROCK"

3. "ROLL" CATCH

*h/t @cassi.niemann and @ucanrow2*

## When?

During the rowing stroke recovery

## What does this mean?

From the finish position, keep your hips/seat in place and allow your shoulders to ROCK forward of your hips. Then allow the seat to ROLL forward to the catch position.

## Why is this important?

This technique sets your body in a stronger position for the catch and maximizes the efficiency of your leg drive.

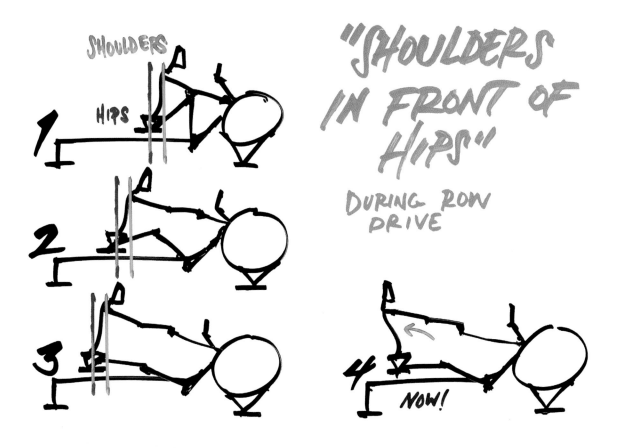

*"SHOULDERS IN FRONT OF HIPS"*
DURING ROW DRIVE

## When?

The drive of the rowing stroke

## What does this mean?

During the drive, keep your shoulders slightly in front of your hips until you've pushed with your legs; then swing your upper body back.

## Why is this important?

This technique allows you to lengthen the stroke and apply a longer drive of power.

# CHAPTER (14)

## SETUP

# BODY PROPORTIONS & SET UPS

| LONG TORSO LONG ARMS | LONG TORSO SHORT ARMS | SHORT TORSO LONG ARMS | SHORT TORSO SHORT ARMS |

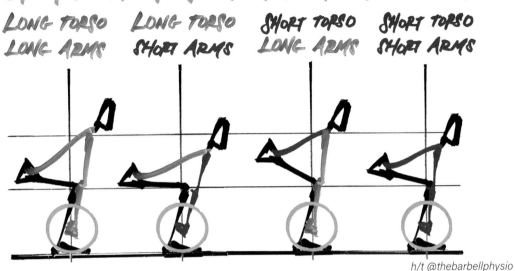

*h/t @thebarbellphysio*

## When?

Deadlift

## What does this mean?

Your relative limb lengths will change how you set up for deadlifts:

- **Long arms** (relative to the trunk/legs): Many of the best deadlifters have long arms, which let an athlete set up higher and reduce the total range of motion the barbell must be lifted. Look at the stick figure on the far left versus the others. The long-arm athlete has a higher hip position in the setup and a more upright torso.

- **Long trunk** (relative to the thigh): Athletes with a short torso (or a relatively long thigh), often see a more forward torso angle relative to the ground. A shorter thigh (or longer torso) means their hips won't be as far behind the barbell as someone with a taller torso.

In general, most athletes deadlift with their shoulders higher than their hips and their hips higher than their knees.

## Why is this important?

Your overall proportions are one piece in the puzzle as to why they move certain ways with the barbell.

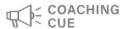
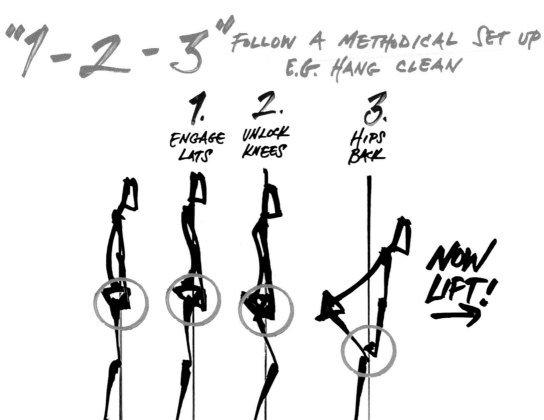

"1-2-3" FOLLOW A METHODICAL SET UP
E.G. HANG CLEAN

1. ENGAGE LATS
2. UNLOCK KNEES
3. HIPS BACK

NOW LIFT!

## When?

Setting up for hang cleans (but can be applied to any setup)

## What does this mean?

Often I see beginner lifters carelessly set up. The result is a weak lift.

For hang cleans, I set up using the following steps:

1. Engage lats

2. Unlock knees

3. Push hips back to the catch position.

## Why is this important?

Following a methodical process each time simplifies the lift and enables you to be in the best start position every time. Regardless of the lift, find your optimal methodical process and use it every time.

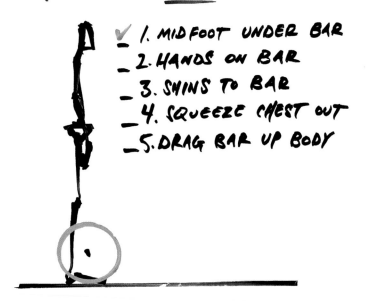

"BE METHODICAL WITH YOUR SET-UP."
— FOLLOW A METHOD EACH TIME —

✓ 1. MIDFOOT UNDER BAR
_ 2. HANDS ON BAR
_ 3. SHINS TO BAR
_ 4. SQUEEZE CHEST OUT
_ 5. DRAG BAR UP BODY

h/t @startingstrength

## When?

Setting up to lift

## What does this mean?

Me: What's the root word of *methodical*?

Students (jokingly): "Meth!"

Me: No, *method*. I want you to be methodical with your setup. Take your time and follow a step-by-step method to get yourself into the best position BEFORE you move the barbell.

## Why is this important?

Being methodical with your setup not only helps with placing you in the best position to lift but also builds body awareness and creates a ritual prior to engaging in a movement.

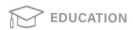 

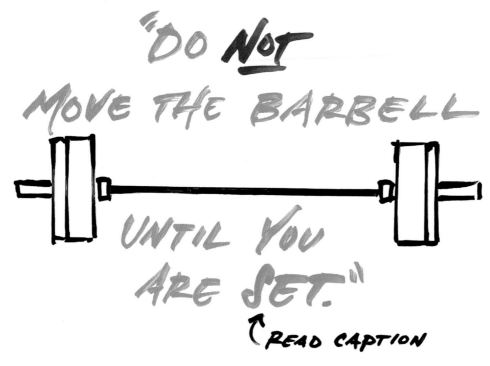

"DO NOT MOVE THE BARBELL UNTIL YOU ARE SET."

↑ READ CAPTION

## When?

Any barbell movement

## What does this mean?

A common error with beginner lifters is their carelessness in rushing the setup for a lift. Take the time to follow these three steps for a successful setup.

1. **Stance:** Set your feet exactly where you want them to be prior to moving the bar. Ninety-nine percent of the time, that means the bar is directly over your mid-foot—approximately hip width for pulling exercises and approximately shoulder width for squatting exercises.

2. **Grip:** Set your hands on the bar exactly where you want prior to moving the bar. The most common grip is hands just outside of your shoulders. Squeeze the bar like you mean it.

3. **Position:** Set your body in position prior to moving the bar. Brace your core. Fix your eyes. Set tension on the bar.

Once you have taken these steps to get set, THEN move the barbell.

## Why is this important?

Being methodical about your setup each time you move the barbell gives you a better start, and a better start leads to a better finish.

# "FREE THROW LINE"

## WHEN SETTING UP FOR A BARBELL MOVEMENT OFF THE GROUND

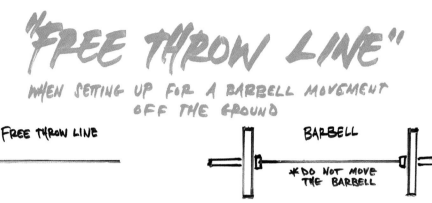
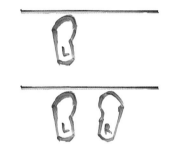
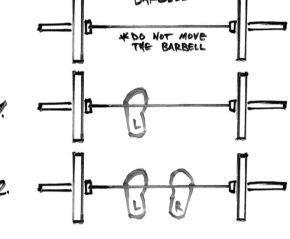

FREE THROW LINE

BARBELL

*DO NOT MOVE THE BARBELL

1.

2.

NOW DRIBBLE THE BALL   3.   NOW HANDS ON THE BAR

## When?

Setting up for a barbell movement off the ground

## What does this mean?

Take a methodical approach to setting up for a barbell movement off the ground just as you would if you were stepping up to the free throw line:

- You do not roll the free throw line back to you. You step up TO the free throw line. In the same way, don't roll the bar back to you. Step up TO the bar.

- You do not shoot the ball until you are ready to shoot. In the same way, do not move the barbell until you are set to lift it.

## Why is this important?

The best athletes in all sports always have a ritual before performing. An established ritual resets your brain.

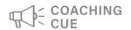

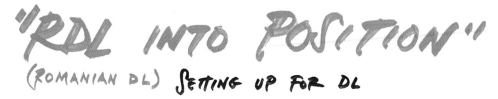

# "RDL INTO POSITION"
## (ROMANIAN DL) SETTING UP FOR DL

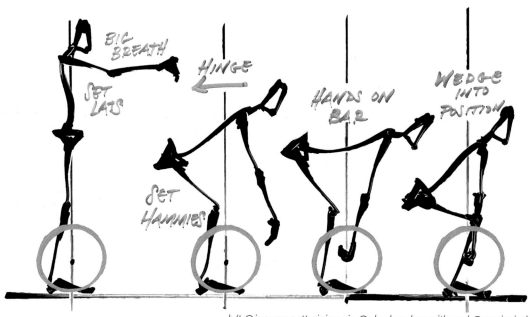

*h/t @juggernauttraining via @chadwesleysmith and @marisainda*

## When?
Setting up for deadlifts, cleans, and snatches

## What does this mean?
Begin your setup from the top down. After you have your feet in position under the bar, hinge back as if you are doing an "air RDL" (Romanian deadlift). Once your hands are on the bar, keep tension through your body and wedge yourself into position.

## Why is this important?
This technique sets tension through your posterior chain and prepares your body to lift.

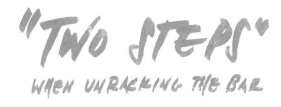

# "TWO STEPS"
## WHEN UNRACKING THE BAR

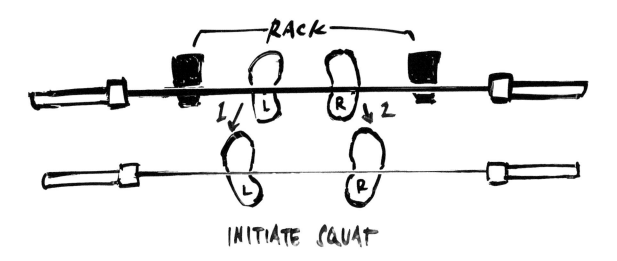

INITIATE SQUAT

## When?

Unracking the bar

## What does this mean?

Try to make a ritual out of unracking the bar:

1.  Set your feet under the bar and in a hip-width stance.

2.  BRACE!

3.  Stand the bar off the rack (do a "mini-squat").

4.  Step one foot back to squat-width stance.

5.  Step the second foot back to squat-width stance.

6.  Initiate the squat.

*NOTE:* Of course *everyone is different* and has (and should have) their own routine/ritual. The idea with this cue is to illustrate the importance of moving with a purpose and being efficient.

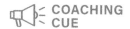
# "UNRACK THE BAR WITH YOUR SHOULDERS!"
## — FRONT RACK MOVEMENTS —

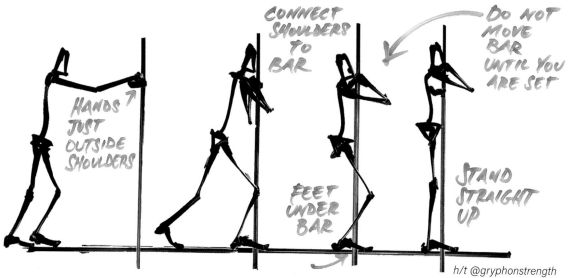

CONNECT SHOULDERS TO BAR

DO NOT MOVE BAR UNTIL YOU ARE SET

HANDS JUST OUTSIDE SHOULDERS

FEET UNDER BAR

STAND STRAIGHT UP

h/t @gryphonstrength

## When?

Front-rack movements

## What does this mean?

You must make a secure connection between your trunk and the barbell to stabilize the bar and create an efficient transfer of power from your lower body.

In an optimal front rack, the barbell sits in the channel between the base of your neck and the rear of your deltoid.

When setting up, establish this connection with the bar in the rack before you unrack it.

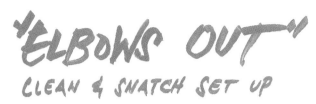
# "ELBOWS OUT"
## CLEAN & SNATCH SET UP

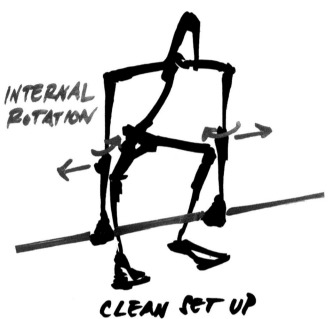

INTERNAL ROTATION

CLEAN SET UP

*h/t @catalystathletics*

## When?
Setup for clean and snatch

## What does this mean?
During the setup for the clean and the snatch, internally rotate your arms so the bony points of your elbows are facing away from your body.

## Why is this important?
Keeping this arm position through the first and second pulls enable you to more easily pull your elbows up and out to the sides during the third pull. Additionally, this position keeps the bar path closer to your body.

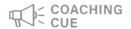
# "KNEES COVER THE BAR"
## SET UP FOR DL, SNATCH, CLEAN

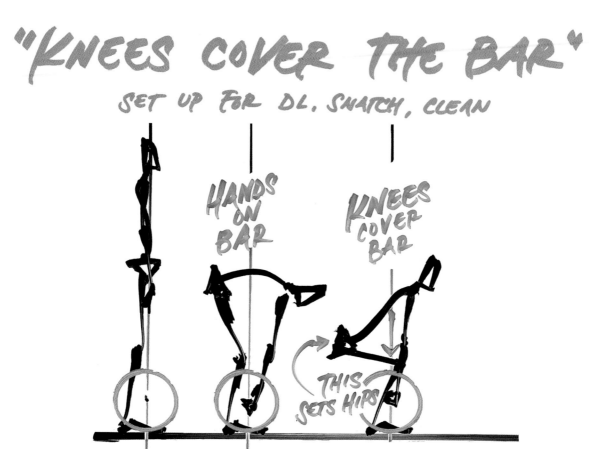

HANDS ON BAR

KNEES COVER BAR

THIS SETS HIPS

## When?

Setting up for a lift from the floor

## What does this mean?

When setting up for deadlift, clean, or snatch variations, your mid-foot should be under the barbell. After you place your hands on the bar, set your hips at the right position by moving your knees forward of the bar ("covering the bar") from your line of sight.

The angle of your back is dependent on your limb length. However, your hips should be higher than your knees, and your shoulders should be higher than your hips.

## Why is this important?

Placing your knees in the right position sets your hips in the right position. Because your hips are the prime movers of lifting the bar from the floor, their position is critical.

# "EYES UP, CHEST OUT"
## SETUP FOR SNATCH/CLEAN

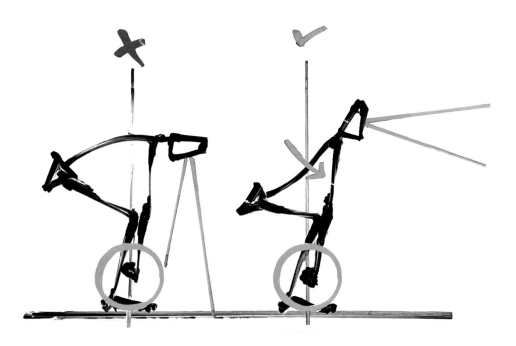

## When?

Setting up for snatch or clean

## What does this mean?

Often when working with beginner lifters, I've noticed that they tend to look "where the action is"—usually at their feet, hands, or the barbell. This places them in a weak position with high hips, lack of engagement through the core, and no visual focus.

## Why is this important?

By setting your eyes on the horizon, you can focus on a single spot throughout the entire lift. By pushing your chest out, you engage your lats and create stiffness throughout your core. A by-product of these two actions usually fixes your hip height and draws your hips into a more powerful position.

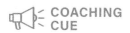

# "LOWER BACK SHIRT WRINKLES"
## DURING DL SETUP

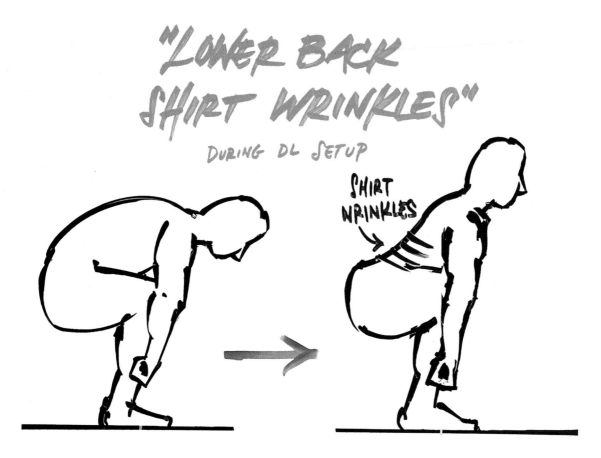

SHIRT WRINKLES

### When?
Deadlift setup

### What does this mean?
During the setup for a deadlift, when you push your chest out, depress your scaps, and engage your lats, wrinkles appear on the lumbar region of your shirt.

### Why is this important?
Although it's impossible for you to see this, mentally visualizing the wrinkles may help you understand the positioning. Additionally, it may help you when you're watching another lifter demonstrating this.

# "SOFT KNEES, HIPS BACK"
## GETTING SET FOR HANG POSITION

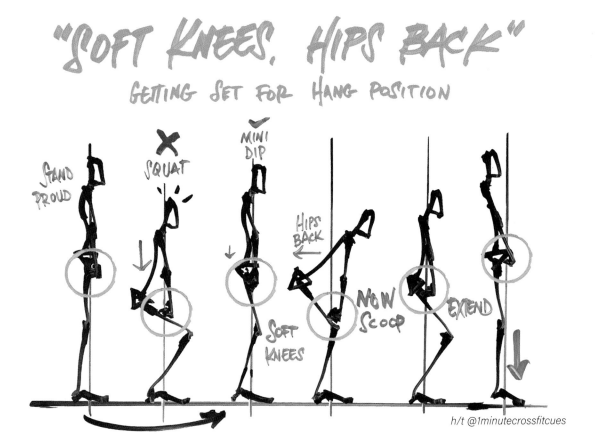

STAND PROUD

X SQUAT

MINI DIP

HIPS BACK

NOW SCOOP

EXTEND

SOFT KNEES

*h/t @1minutecrossfitcues*

## When?

Setting up for the hang position

## What does this mean?

I often see beginners squatting as they get set in the hang position. Squatting places you in an imbalanced position with the majority of the tension in your quads.

Instead, from a standing position, put a slight bend in your knee and then hinge your hips back.

## Why is this important?

Hinging your hips back efficiently places the tension in the powerful posterior chain and primes your system for aggressive extension.

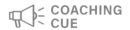
# "GET TIGHT FIRST"

### SETTING UP FOR BACK SQUAT

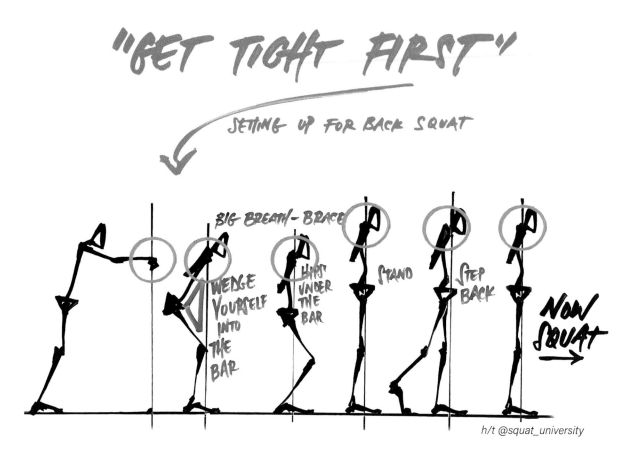

BIG BREATH - BRACE

WEDGE YOURSELF INTO THE BAR

HIPS UNDER THE BAR

STAND

STEP BACK

NOW SQUAT

*h/t @squat_university*

## When?

Setting up for back squat

## What does this mean?

To get the most out of your positioning, take full advantage of the bar being "weightless" when it is on the rack. Take your time from the ground up to get in the right position and build tremendous stiffness throughout your core *before* you unrack the bar. Once you're set, *then* unrack the weight.

## Why is this important?

Once you start your rep, it's challenging to adjust your positioning. You need to have your positioning correct before you start.

# "EYES ON THE HORIZON"

## SETUP FOR SNATCH & CLEAN

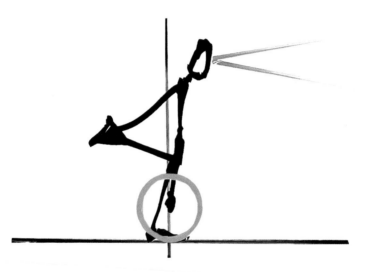

### When?
Setup position for snatch or clean

### What does this mean?
When setting up for the snatch or clean, look to the horizon.

### Why is this important?
When you look at the floor, your chest naturally points toward the floor, making the mobility requirements for you to keep the bar above your head greater. Looking at the horizon helps keep your chest upright and provides you with a focal point throughout the entire movement.

# CHAPTER 15

## SHOULDER TO OVERHEAD

# "HEAD THROUGH THE WINDOW"

## WHEN SUPPORTING WEIGHT OVERHEAD

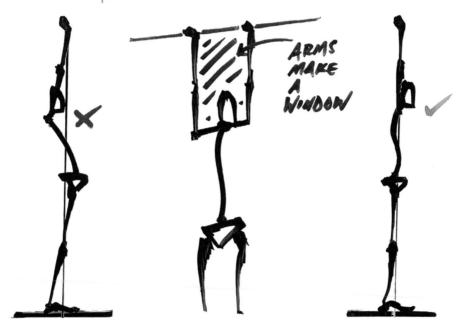

ARMS MAKE A WINDOW

## When?

Overhead positions

## What does this mean?

Cue the athlete to push their head through the "window" that their arms make when pressing overhead.

## Why is this important?

Pushing the head forward may help the athlete finish the lift by placing the weight (bar, kettlebell, body weight) in line with their shoulders and hips.

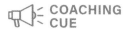

# COACHING CUE

# "MAKE AN ICE CREAM CONE"
### —HAND/WRIST POSITION: SNATCH & JERK —

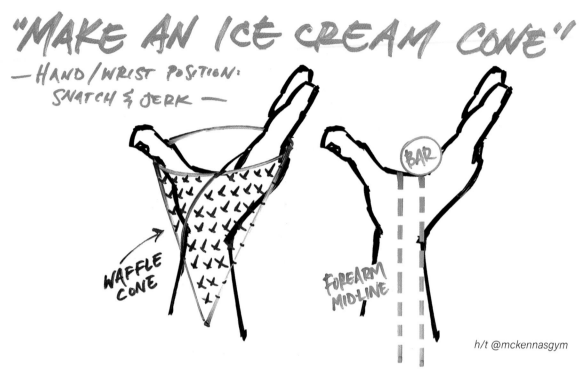

WAFFLE CONE

FOREARM MIDLINE

BAR

*h/t @mckennasgym*

### When?

Hand/wrist position in jerk and snatch

### What does this mean?

The hand/wrist position in the jerk and snatch should mimic the shape of an ice cream cone, with the bar being a scoop of ice cream. Extend your wrist so your palm points up. The bar should rest in the palm of your hand, slightly behind the midline of your forearm.

This basic position meets a few pretty simple criteria:

- The barbell is over your forearm, ideally slightly behind your midline.
- Your wrist is extended (not neutral) but not hyperextended.
- The heel of your palm is pointing somewhat toward the ceiling.

### Why is this important?

A neutral wrist position is unstable and creates an equal tendency to move in both directions (forward and back). It also places more strain on your wrist.

*Note:* Read more in the article "Hand & Wrist Position in the Snatch & Jerk" from @catalystathletics.

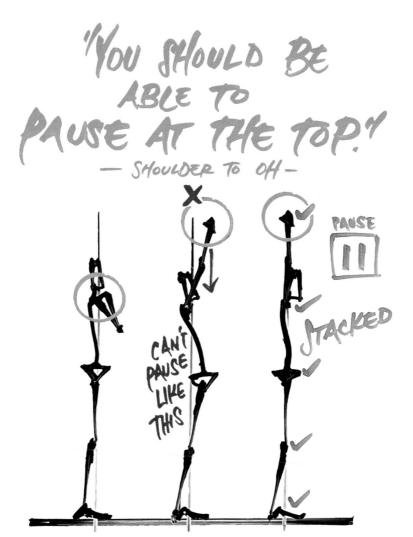

"YOU SHOULD BE ABLE TO PAUSE AT THE TOP."

— SHOULDER TO OH —

## When?

Any shoulder to overhead press

## What does this mean?

An overhead rep (even a KB swing) is complete when a lockout takes place not only with your shoulders and arms but also your hips and legs.

## Why is this important?

When you do this properly, these joints should be stacked on top of each other, allowing the movement to pause and creating a stable position.

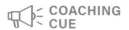
"HOW FAR SHOULD I DIP?"
"10% OF YOUR HEIGHT"
— PUSH PRESS, JERK —

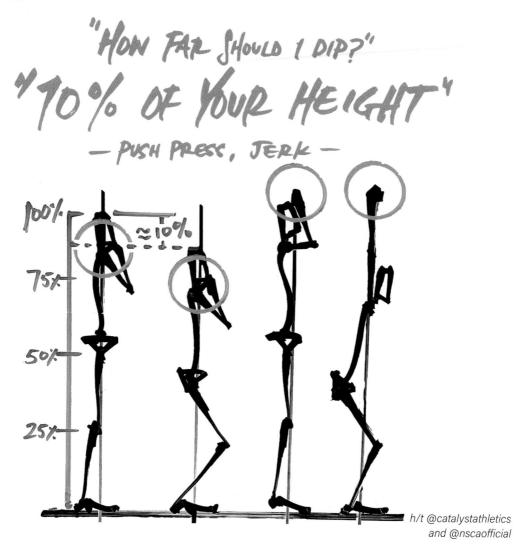

h/t @catalystathletics
and @nscaofficial

## When?

During the dip of the push press or jerk

## What does this mean?

The depth of the dip during the push press or jerk should be about 10 percent of your height.

# "CONTROL THE DIP"
## DURING PUSH PRESS & JERK

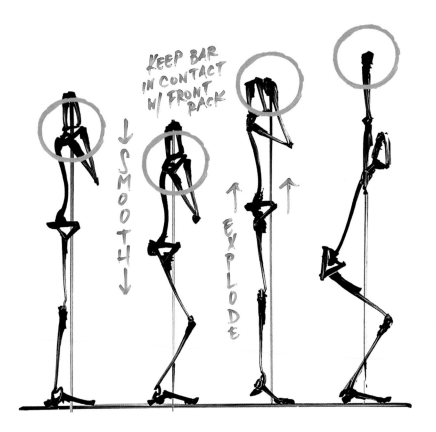

KEEP BAR IN CONTACT W/ FRONT RACK

SMOOTH

EXPLODE

## When?

During the push press or jerk

## What does this mean?

A common error is dipping too quickly and losing connection of the bar in the front rack. Keep the dip smooth and controlled and stay connected with the bar.

## Why is this important?

Controlling the dip creates a stable and smooth transfer of power.

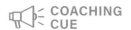

# "CORKSCREW YOUR KNEES"
## DURING DIP OF JERK / PP

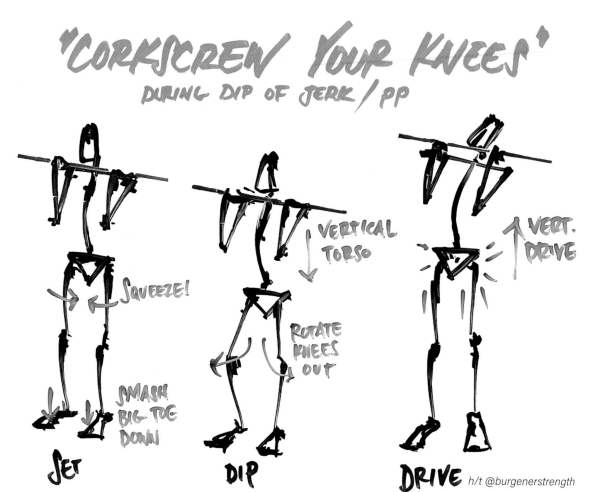

SQUEEZE!

SMASH BIG TOE DOWN

**SET**

VERTICAL TORSO

ROTATE KNEES OUT

**DIP**

VERT. DRIVE

**DRIVE** h/t @burgenerstrength

## When?

During the dip of the jerk or push press

## What does this mean?

Anchor your feet by smashing your big toes into the ground. Squeeze your inner thighs together. Rotate your knees out ("corkscrew your knees"). You should feel your glutes firing.

Unlock your knees into a shallow dip, keeping your torso upright. Then drive hard, squeezing your quads and glutes to create hip and knee extension.

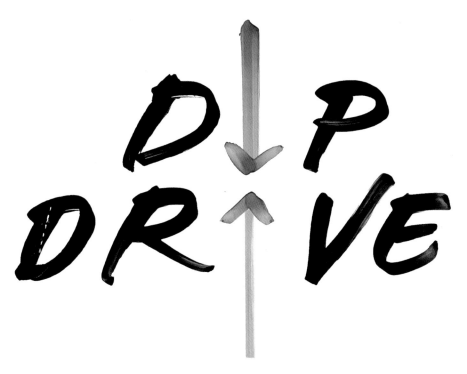

# DIP
# DRIVE

## KEEP IT VERTICAL FOR PUSH PRESS/JERK

### When?
Push press/jerk

### What does this mean?
This illustration may help remind you to keep the orientation of the torso vertical during the dip and drive of the push press/jerk.

### Why is this important?
For the push press and push jerk, you want the bar to go up. The dip and drive are vertical movements—down then up. Any lateral displacement is wasted energy and leads to a less efficient bar path.

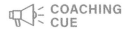

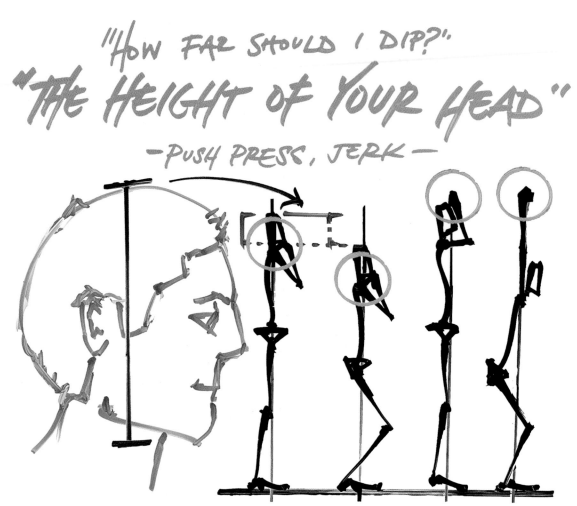

"How far should I dip?"
"The Height of Your Head"
— Push Press, Jerk —

## When?

Knowing how far to go during the dip of the push press or jerk

## What does this mean?

The average head is approximately 10 percent of the person's height. This is the recommended distance to dip during the push press or jerk.

# "HIPS TO HEELS"
## — DURING THE DIP — OF PUSH PRESS/JERK

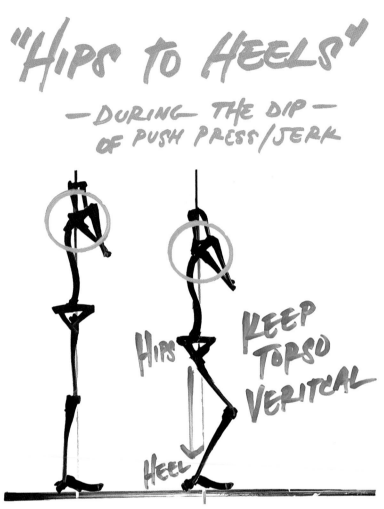

HIPS

KEEP TORSO VERTICAL

HEEL

## When?
During the dip of the push press or jerk

## What does this mean?
Keep your shoulders, hips, and ankles in a straight vertical line throughout the dip (and drive).

## Why is this important?
Maintaining straight alignment keeps your balance over the foot and ensures the bar trajectory is up and slightly back.

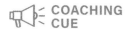
# "IN A PHONE BOOTH"
## —PUSH PRESS, PUSH JERK—

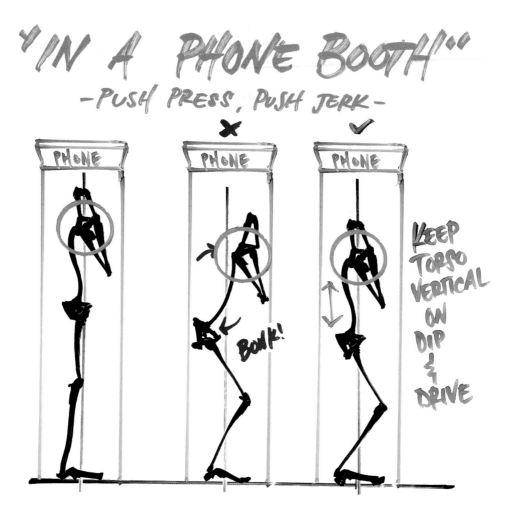

## When?

Push press and push jerk

## What does this mean?

During the dip and drive of the push press or push jerk, your torso should remain vertical. You can imagine you are in a phone booth. If you lean forward or backward, you'll hit the walls. Keep your torso upright when dipping and driving.

## Why is this important?

During the push press and push jerk, you want the bar to go up. For the bar to go up, you need to apply force in the opposite direction: down. Leaning forward or backward leads to wasted movement as the bar and your hips drift laterally. Keep that force moving in a straight vertical line.

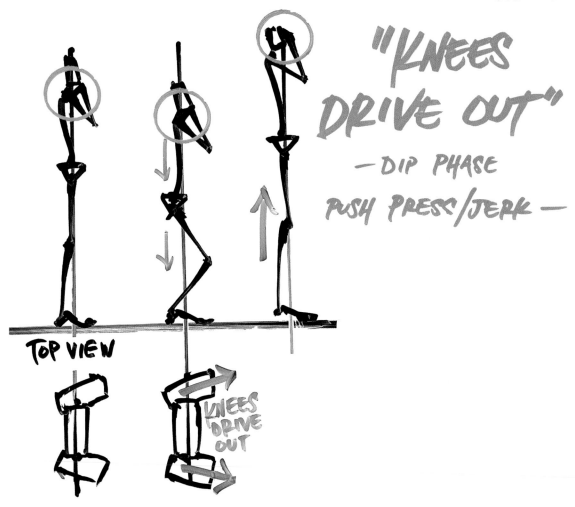

# "KNEES DRIVE OUT"

## — DIP PHASE PUSH PRESS/JERK —

TOP VIEW

KNEES DRIVE OUT

## When?

During the dip of the push press or jerk

## What does this mean?

Stand with your feet approximately hip-width apart with your toes slightly turned out. With the bar in the jerk rack position, initiate the dip phase by keeping your torso vertical and driving your knees out in the same direction as your feet.

## Why is this important?

This technique helps keep your torso vertical and engages the powerful glutes for the drive upward.

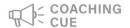

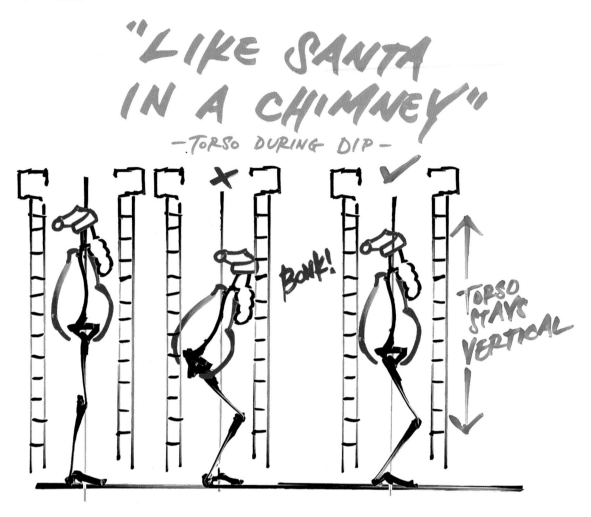

"LIKE SANTA IN A CHIMNEY"

—TORSO DURING DIP—

## When?

Torso angle during the dip

## What does this mean?

In order for Santa to go up and down a chimney, he has to keep his torso vertical. Otherwise, he'll hit his head or hips against the bricks.

Similarly, during the dip and drive of the push press or push jerk, keep your torso vertical.

# "LOAD THE SPRING"
## — PUSH PRESS / JERK —

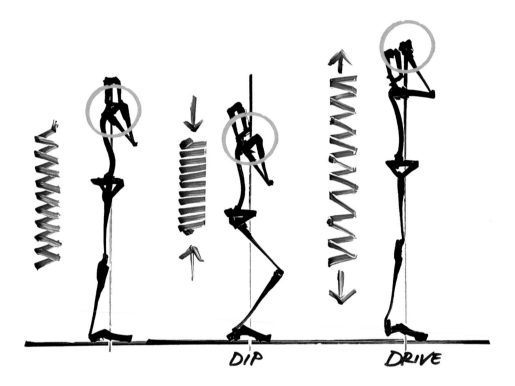

DIP          DRIVE

## When?

Push press and jerk

## What does this mean?

The dip and drive of the push press or jerk can be described as loading and extending. As the torso dips straight down, power is loaded in the legs. During the extension of the legs, power is transferred through the torso into the bar.

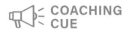
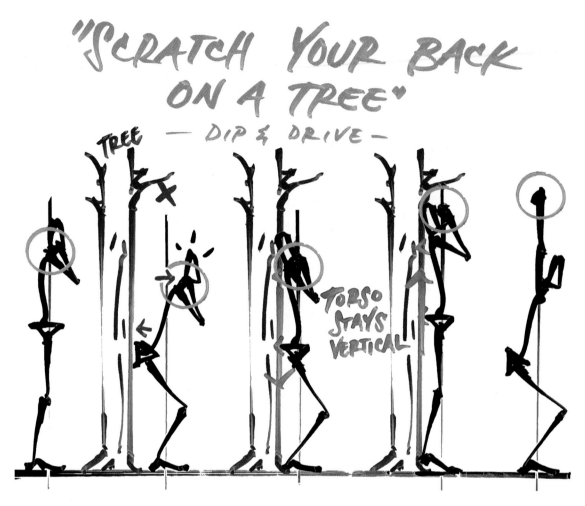

"SCRATCH YOUR BACK ON A TREE"
— DIP & DRIVE —

TREE

TORSO STAYS VERTICAL

## When?

Push press and push jerk dip and drive

## What does this mean?

During the dip and drive of the push press or push jerk, keep your torso vertical, as if you are scratching your back up and down against a tree.

# "SLIDE UP AND DOWN A WALL"
## DURING DIP & DRIVE

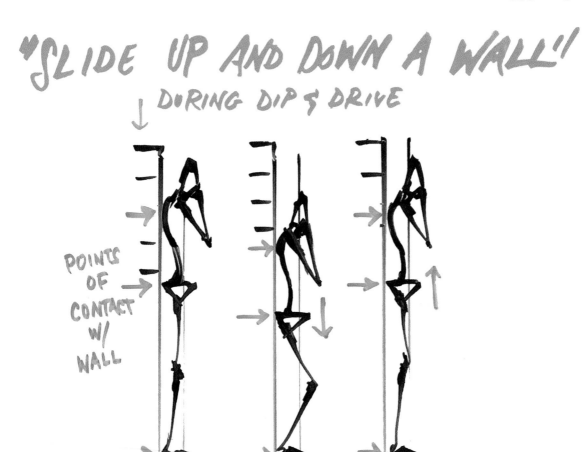

POINTS
OF
CONTACT
W/
WALL

### When?
Dip and drive of the push press and jerk

### What does this mean?
Your torso should move up and down in a vertical line during the dip and drive of the push press and jerk.

This movement pattern is identical to standing with your hips, shoulders, and heels against a wall. Try this as a tactile cue. If all three points stay in contact with the wall during the dip and drive, the movement pattern is vertical.

### Why is this important?
Staying vertical keeps the weight balanced over your mid-foot.

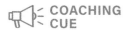
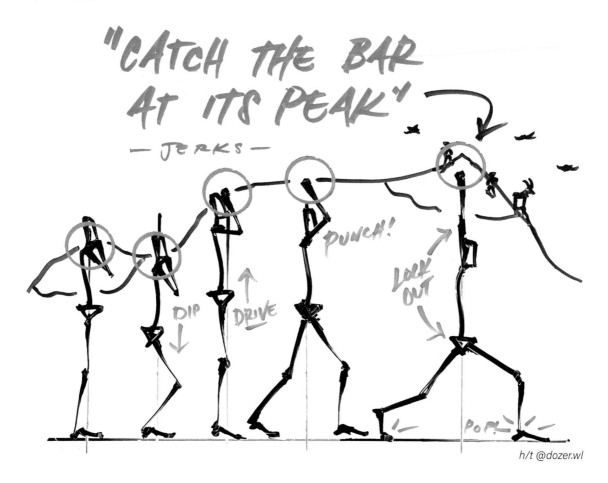

"CATCH THE BAR AT ITS PEAK"

— JERKS —

DIP
DRIVE
PUNCH!
LOCK OUT
POP

h/t @dozer.wl

## When?

Jerk

## What does this mean?

When the bar is at the peak of its path, it's "weightless" for an extremely brief moment before beginning its trajectory back down. The closer you can receive the bar to that peak with a stable stance, rigid torso, and locked-out arms, the easier the lift will be.

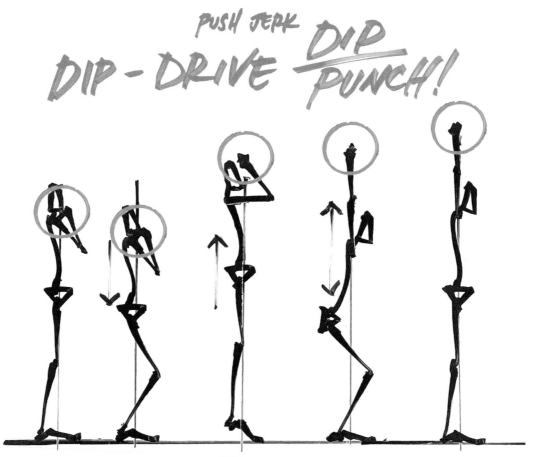

PUSH JERK
## DIP - DRIVE ~~DIP PUNCH!~~

**When?**

Push jerk

**What does this mean?**

A common error I've noticed when working with novice lifters is the timing sequence when locking out the barbell overhead.

This may incorrectly be
**Dip→Drive→Punch→Dip→**

Or
**Dip→Drive→Dip→Punch**

It should be
**Dip→Drive→Dip/punch**

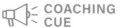
# PUSH JERK
# DIP - DRIVE - SIT!

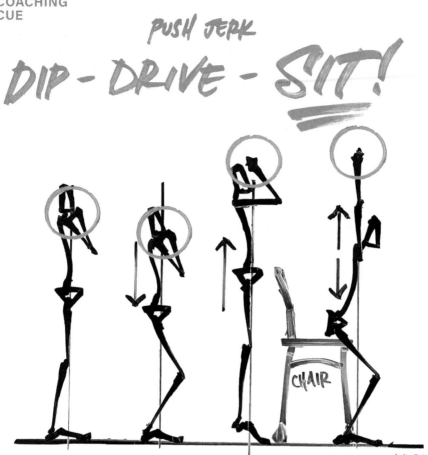

*h/t @1minutecrossfitcues*

### When?

Push jerk

### What does this mean?

A common cue for the movement sequence of the jerk is to "dip–drive–dip." However, this does not describe the proper torso position for the athlete during the receive.

Dipping means the hips stay under your shoulders. Instead, your hips should sit back, similar to receiving a power clean. This movement pattern resembles a squat, not a dip.

### Why is this important?

Receiving the bar in the overhead position with a dip unevenly loads the quads rather than the powerful posterior chain. Sitting in a partial squat is a more balanced and powerful position when you're supporting a load overhead.

# "LEGS LIKE ROOF TRUSSES"
## –SPLIT JERK RECEIVE–

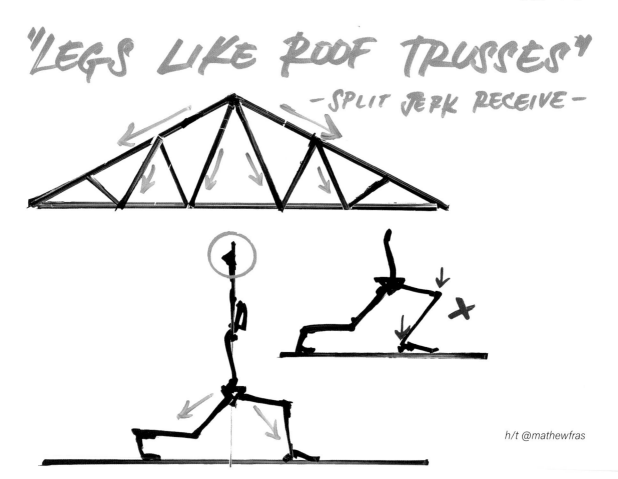

*h/t @mathewfras*

## When?

Split jerk receive

## What does this mean?

Trusses are built to support the weight of the roof. The braces are designed so they angle out, away from the center. Similarly, the angle of your legs is very important to support both your bodyweight and the weight of the bar.

To create a supportive truss with your legs, your leading shin should be vertical, with your knee directly above your ankle. Your trailing leg should be slightly bent. Your feet should share equal pressure.

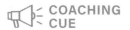
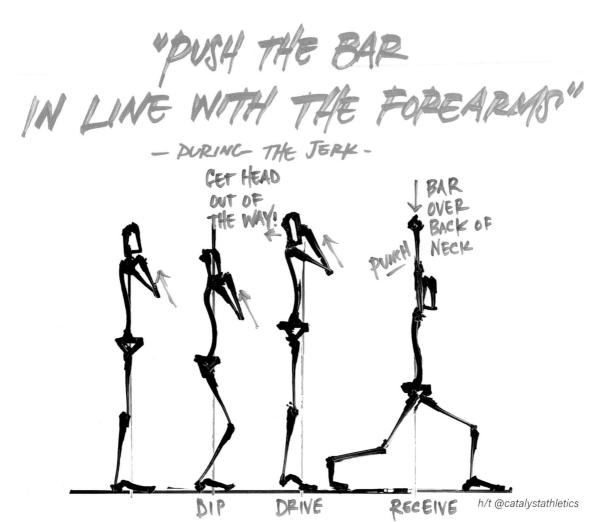

"PUSH THE BAR IN LINE WITH THE FOREARMS"

— DURING THE JERK —

GET HEAD OUT OF THE WAY!

↓ BAR OVER BACK OF NECK

PUNCH

DIP    DRIVE    RECEIVE    *h/t @catalystathletics*

## When?

Jerk

## What does this mean?

During the jerk rack position, your upper arms should roughly be in the five o'clock position when viewed from the side. When you initiate the drive or jerk, aim to push the bar in the same angle as your forearms. The result will be the lockout occurring directly above your neck.

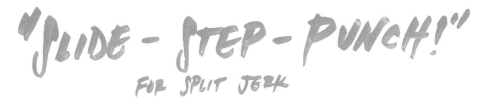

# "SLIDE - STEP - PUNCH!"

## FOR SPLIT JERK

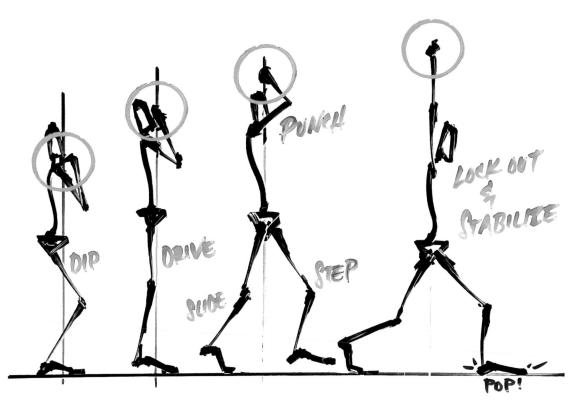

DIP

DRIVE

SLIDE

STEP

PUNCH

LOCK OUT & STABILIZE

POP!

## When?

Split jerk

## What does this mean?

Immediately following the extension of your hips and knees during the drive, the bar is launched from the front-rack position.

You slide your rear foot back, step your front foot forward, and punch the bar overhead.

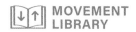
# "JERK RECEIVING POSITIONS"

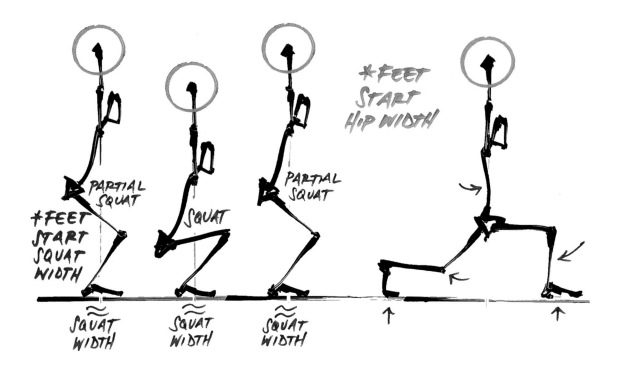

*FEET START SQUAT WIDTH

PARTIAL SQUAT

SQUAT

PARTIAL SQUAT

*FEET START HIP WIDTH

SQUAT WIDTH

SQUAT WIDTH

SQUAT WIDTH

## Points of Performance

**Setup:**

- Hip-width stance
- Grip width just outside of shoulders
- Elbows slightly in front of bar
- Full grip on bar

**Movement:**

- Dip your torso straight down.
- Extend your hips and legs rapidly and then press under.
- Drive your heels down until your hips and legs fully extend.
- Receive the bar in split position.
- Bring your feet together one at a time.
- Stabilize the bar over the middle of your foot.
- The lift is complete when both feet are together with full arm, hip, and knee extension.

# "STAY IN YOUR LANE"
## STANCE DURING LUNGE / SPLIT VARIATIONS

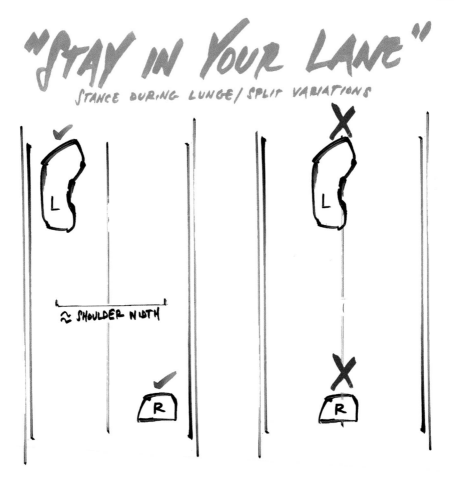

## When?

Establishing split stance width

## What does this mean?

When establishing a stable stance for the split jerk or lunge, the distance between your feet should be approximately shoulder width.

Cue your athletes to keep each of their feet in their own lane, approximately shoulder-width distance apart.

## Why is this important?

A common error with beginning lifters is to shorten this width during the step, which creates a less stable stance.

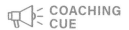
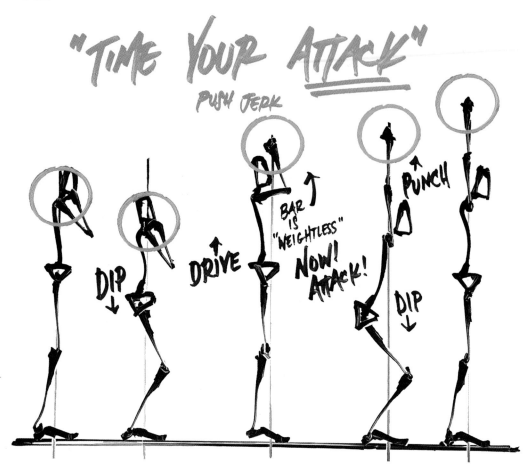

## When?
Push jerk

## What does this mean?
During the explosive initial drive of the jerk, the bar reaches its maximum velocity and then experiences a split second of "weightlessness," typically just above your head.

At that brief moment, "time your attack" on the bar with an aggressive dip and punch on the bar. Receive the bar with locked out arms and a partial squat.

## Why is this important?
The timing of this sequence is crucial to maximize the efficiency of the movement.

# "HIPS START, ARMS FINISH"
## — PUSH PRESS —

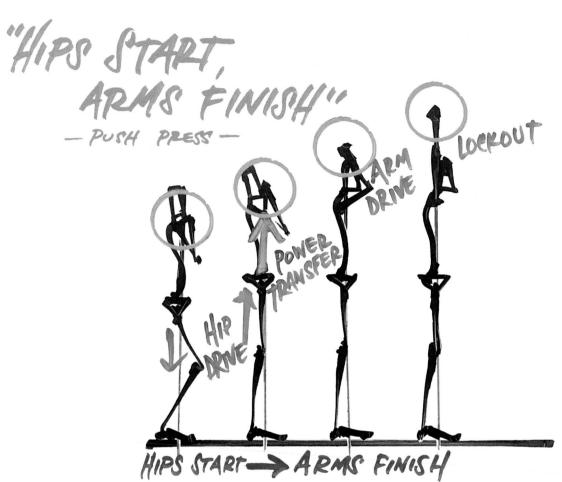

LOCKOUT

ARM DRIVE

POWER TRANSFER

HIP DRIVE

HIPS START → ARMS FINISH

## When?

Push press

## What does this mean?

During the push press, vertical power is initiated with an explosive hip/knee extension. Power transfers through the torso and into the bar. The moment the hips and knees extend, the arms continue the vertical power through lockout.

## Why is this important?

Efficient movement occurs in a wave of contraction from the core outward to the extremities. A common beginner error during the push press is initiating the press with the arms prior to the extension of the hips. Doing so cuts the power short from the hips.

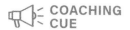
# "OPEN UP YOUR KNEE JOINT"
## PUSH PRESS

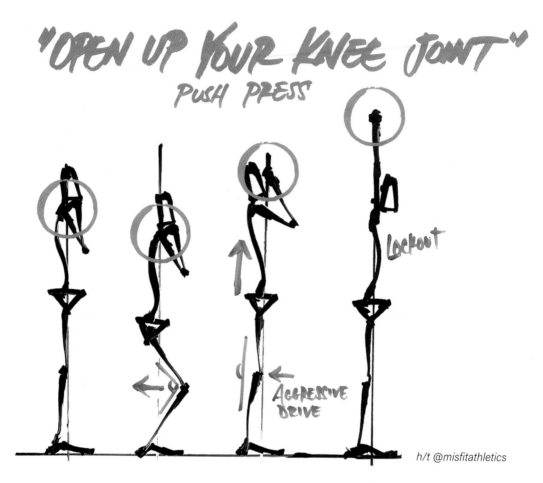

Lockout

AGGRESSIVE
DRIVE

*h/t @misfitathletics*

### When?
Driving out of the push press

### What does this mean?
During the upward drive of the push press, you obviously want aggressive extension through the hip. If you have problems throwing your hips forward, focus on aggressively opening the knee joint.

### Why is this important?
It is impossible to drive the torso vertically without extending your knees.

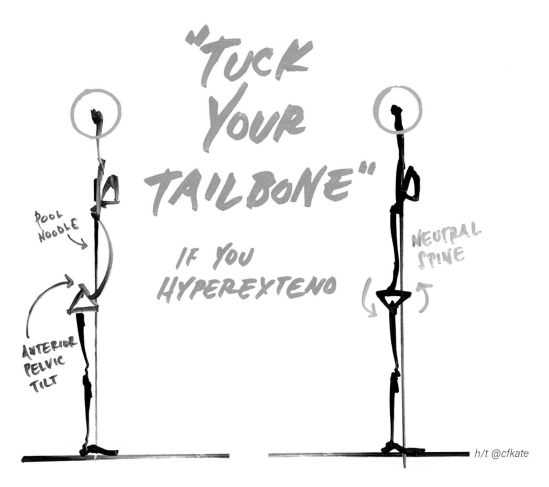

"TUCK
YOUR
TAILBONE"

IF YOU
HYPEREXTEND

POOL
NOODLE

ANTERIOR
PELVIC
TILT

NEUTRAL
SPINE

*h/t @cfkate*

## When?

Maintaining a neutral spine during both dynamic and static movements

## What does this mean?

If you are someone who hyperextends your spine, focus on "tucking your tailbone."

Hyperextension is a result of unbalanced engagement through your core, specifically loose glutes and abs. When this happens, your pelvis tilts forward and everything up the chain is unstacked.

Regain a strong posture by contracting your glutes and abs (tucking your tailbone). This will bring your pelvis and spine back to a stacked, neutral position.

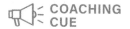
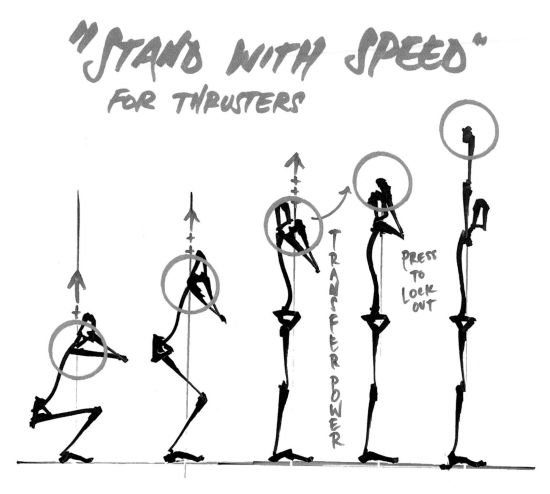

# "STAND WITH SPEED" FOR THRUSTERS

TRANSFER POWER

PRESS TO LOCK OUT

## When?

Thrusters

## What does this mean?

As you drive into extension of your hips and knees, "stand with speed," transferring power through the front rack and into the push press.

Think of the front rack as a launch pad for the barbell and the momentum from the front squat drives seamlessly into pressing the bar overhead.

# "ELBOWS DOWN"
## — PRIOR TO DRIVING BAR UP —
## FOR OHS, DROP SNATCH, SNATCH BALANCE

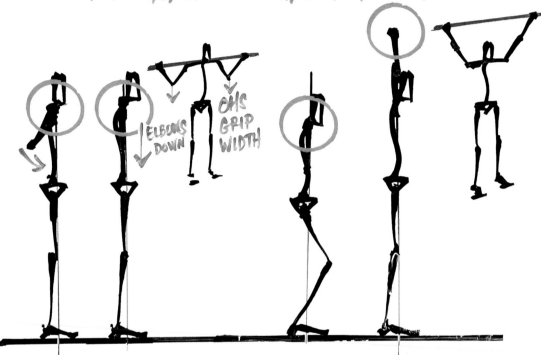

ELBOWS DOWN

OHS GRIP WIDTH

## When?

Setup to drive the bar up into the overhead squat position

## What does this mean?

If the bar is going *up* (for the overhead squat position), the elbows should point *down*.

## Why is this important?

A common beginner error is to allow the elbows to drift behind the bar before dipping and driving the bar overhead. In terms of biomechanics, the most advantageous position for a joint to extend is in line with the object being moved.

# CHAPTER ⑯

## SNATCH AND CLEAN

# THE SNATCH

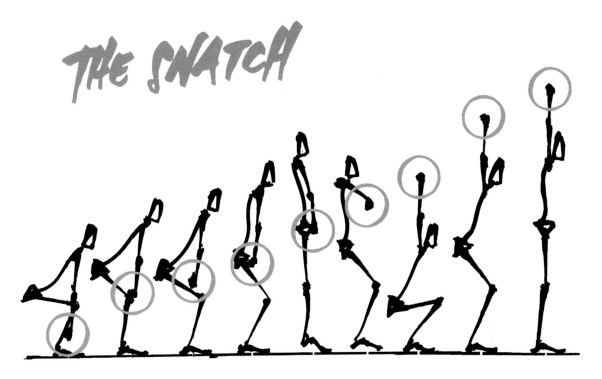

## Points of Performance

### Setup:

- Hip-width stance
- Hands placed at width for overhead squat with hook grip on the bar
- Shoulders slightly in front of the bar

### Movement:

- Maintain the lumbar curve.
- Raise your hips and shoulders at the same rate and then extend your hips rapidly.
- Shrug your shoulders and then pull under with your arms.
- Receive the bar at the bottom of an overhead squat.

The movement is complete at full hip, knee, and arm extension with the bar over the middle of your foot.

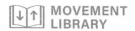
# THE CLEAN

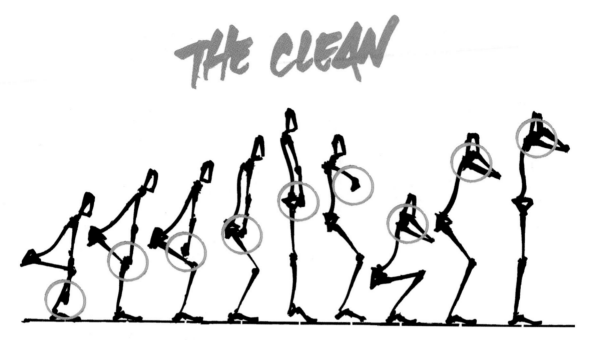

## Points of Performance

### Setup:

- Hip-width stance
- Hands about one thumb's distance from hips
- Hook grip on the bar
- Shoulders slightly in front of the bar

### Movement:

- Maintain your spine's lumbar curve.
- Your hips and shoulders rise at the same rate.
- Keep your heels down and arms straight until your hips and legs extend.
- Extend your hips rapidly.
- Shrug your shoulders and then pull under with your arms.
- Receive the bar at the bottom of a front squat.
- The movement is complete at full hip and knee extension with the bar in the rack position.

# HANG POWER CLEAN

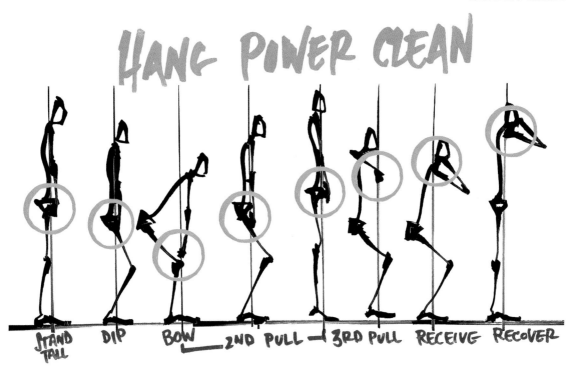

STAND TALL    DIP    BOW    2ND PULL    3RD PULL    RECEIVE    RECOVER

## Points of Performance

**Setup:**

- Hip-width stance
- Grip width is a thumb's width from your thigh
- Hook grip
- Neutral spine maintained

**Movement:**

- Deadlift the bar to the hang position.
- Hinge at the hip and maintain a neutral spine as you lower the bar to the prescribed height:
  - **High-hang:** Upper thigh
  - **Mid-hang:** Mid-thigh
  - **Hang:** Top of knee caps
  - **Knee:** Bar at knee caps
  - **Below knee:** Bar just below knees
- Extend your hips and knees rapidly.
- Keep your heels down until your hips and legs extend.
- Shrug your shoulders and then pull under with your arms.
- Receive the bar in a partial front squat.

The movement is complete at full hip and knee extension with the bar in the front-rack position.

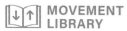
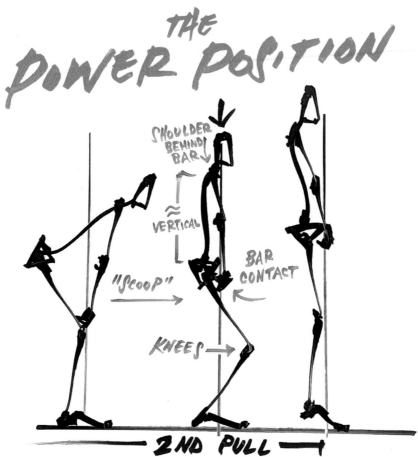

## Points of Performance

- The position occurs during the second pull at the end of the "scoop."
- Your knees are forward.
- Your trunk is approximately vertical.
- Your shoulders are slightly behind the bar.
- The bar is in contact with your body (your hips for a snatch or between your upper thigh and hips for a clean).

# "1 KILO PLATE TOSS"
## TIMING THE CLEAN/SNATCH RECEIVE

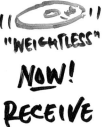

"WEIGHTLESS"

**NOW!**

**RECEIVE**

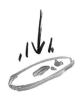

TOO LATE

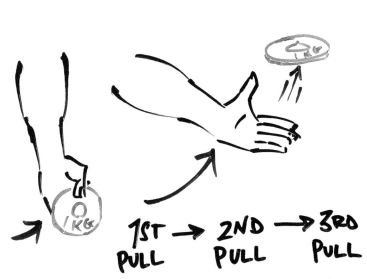

1ST PULL → 2ND PULL → 3RD PULL

### When?
Teaching the timing of the receive for the clean and snatch

### What does this mean?
Take a small-change plate and gently toss it into the air. Notice there is a split-second moment when it is weightless before it begins to drop.

The same thing happens during the clean and snatch. At the end of the second pull, there is a split-second moment when the bar is weightless. It is at that point that you need to receive the bar.

### Why is this important?
Missing this timing will result in the bar crashing down or a missed lift.

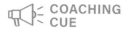
# "ARMS & SHOULDERS CREATE A PENDULUM"

## TO FEEL IF YOU ARE OVER THE BAR.

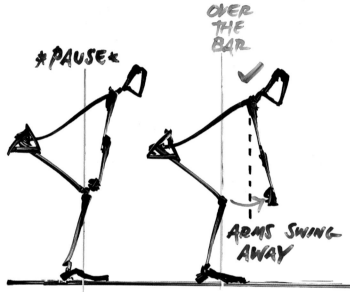

*PAUSE*

OVER
THE
BAR ✓

ARMS SWING
AWAY

*h/t @catalystathletics*

## When?

To feel if you are staying over the bar

## What does this mean?

The weight wants to hang directly below your shoulders. If your shoulders are in front of the bar, the bar wants to move away from your body.

## Why is this important?

During the first and second pulls of the clean or snatch, you should keep your shoulders slightly in front of the bar. This enables you to keep the bar close to your body through the extension of your hips and knees. Additionally, this position forces you to engage your upper back and powerful lats, connecting your body to the bar.

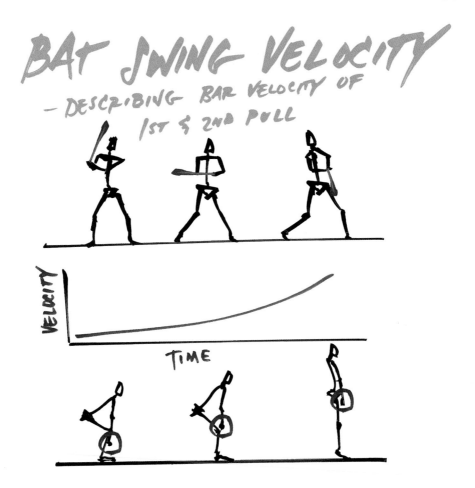

# BAT SWING VELOCITY
## — DESCRIBING BAR VELOCITY OF 1ST & 2ND PULL

## When?

Describing bar velocity for the first and second pulls of the clean and snatch

## What does this mean?

As a batter swings the bat toward the ball, the bat head increases in velocity in a positive slope. Similarly, as the lifter separates the bar from the ground through the first and second pulls, the bar velocity increases in a positive slope.

This cue is most appropriate for an athlete who

- Yanks the bar off the ground (0 to 100mph!)
- Keeps a constant bar speed from ground to receiving position

*Coaching tip:* Identifying similarities between movements in different sports may help your athlete gain a better understanding of their body.

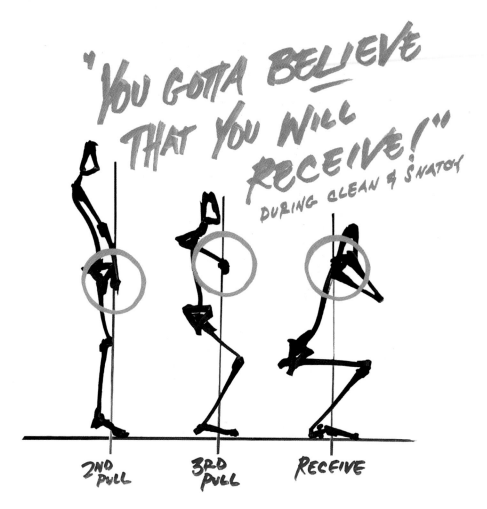

"YOU GOTTA BELIEVE THAT YOU WILL RECEIVE!"

DURING CLEAN & SNATCH

2ND PULL          3RD PULL          RECEIVE

## When?

Snatch and clean

## What does this mean?

Your mental perspective during the clean and snatch must be of the utmost confidence. You must believe in yourself that you will receive the bar.

## Why is this important?

If you doubt yourself, you will likely hesitate. If you hesitate, the bar speed will stall, and the bar will win.

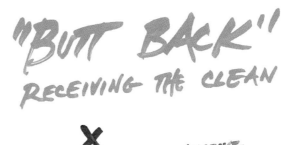

# "BUTT BACK"
## RECEIVING THE CLEAN

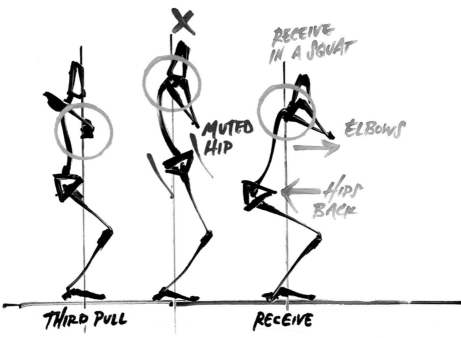

RECEIVE
IN A SQUAT

MUTED
HIP

ELBOWS

HIPS
BACK

THIRD PULL

RECEIVE

## When?

Receiving the clean

## What does this mean?

You should receive the clean in a strong, balanced squat position, with your hips behind your shoulders and mid-foot.

## Why is this important?

A common error in the clean is receiving the bar with a muted hip, resulting in a decrease in stability, balance, and power. This posture is the result of the legs compensating for the hips' failure—specifically, using leg extension to compensate for weak or nonexistent hip extension.

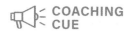
**COACHING CUE**

# "CHECK THE M.E.T.H.O.D., MAN."

**M.** UST
**E.** XTEND
**T.** HE
**H.** IPS
**O.** N
**D.** RIVE

- 2ND PULL -

## When?
Second pull of clean and snatch

## What does this mean?
If you need a helpful reminder to fully extend your hips through the second pull of the clean and snatch, you can use this cue, which references the Wu-Tang Clan song "Method Man." It's an acronym using the letters in *method*:

M: Must
E: Extend
T: The
H: Hips
O: On
D: Drive

# "CLOSE ENOUGH TO SMELL IT"
## BAR PATH DURING 3RD PULL OF SNATCH

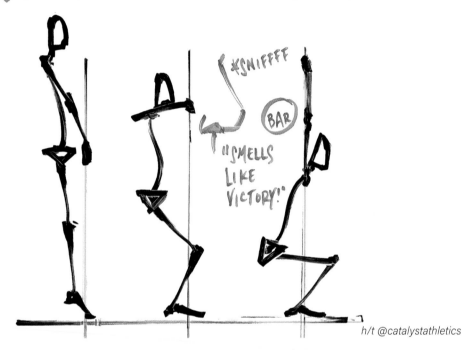

#SNIFFFF

BAR

"SMELLS LIKE VICTORY!"

*h/t @catalystathletics*

## When?

Bar path during the snatch

## What does this mean?

As the bar passes your face during the third pull of the snatch, keep it close enough to smell it.

## Why is this important?

The third pull of the snatch is when you pull your body under the bar and into the receive position. It is during this phase that the bar passes your face, and you push the bar into the locked-out position overhead. The further the bar is away from your face, the less efficient this movement is.

"If you can't smell the bar as it's passing your face, keep it closer."

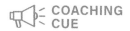
# C.R.E.A.M.
# CLEANS
# REQUIRE
# EXPLOSIVE
# ACCURATE
# MOVEMENT

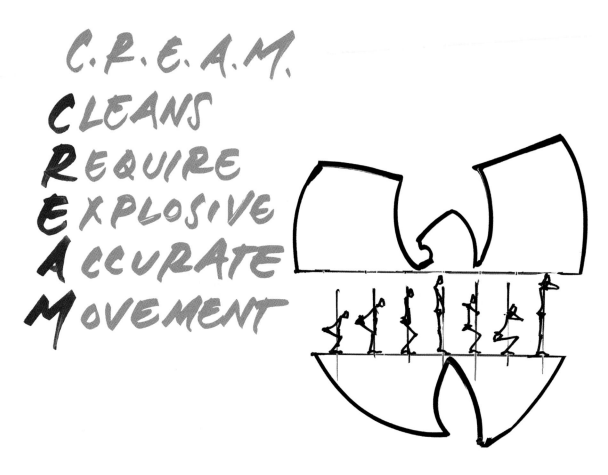

## When?

Cleans and snatches

## What does this mean?

This cue may help you understand the importance of being explosive and aggressive (AND accurate) during the clean and snatch. It references the Wu-Tang Clan song "C.R.E.A.M." and is an acronym of the word.

C: Cleans (and snatches)
R: Require
E: Explosive
A: Aggressive (or Accurate as suggested by @arnondicus)
M: Movement

# "FOOT PRESSURE DICTATES TORSO ANGLE"

## - SNATCH & CLEAN -

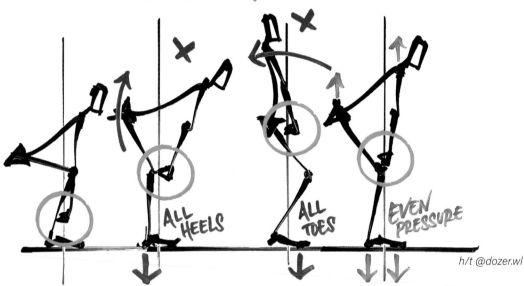

ALL HEELS

ALL TOES

EVEN PRESSURE

*h/t @dozer.wl*

### When?

Snatch and clean

### What does this mean?

During the first and second pulls of the snatch, if all your weight is in your heels the likely result is your hips drive up too quickly. If all of your weight is in your toes, the result is that your shoulders rise too quickly.

### Why is this important?

If you put *even* weight throughout your whole foot during the first and second pulls, your torso angle stays consistent and evenly balanced.

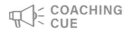 

# "HALF A HEART"
## PATH OF SHOULDERS DURING CLEAN/SNATCH

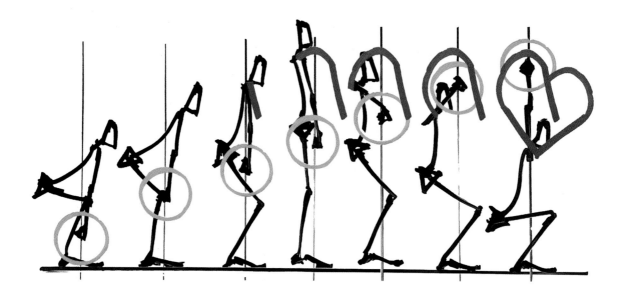

### When?
Clean and snatch

### What does this mean?
For both the clean and the snatch, in order for the bar to travel vertically in a straight path, the shoulders must move in a half heart–shaped path.

# "HIPS MOVE LIKE AN UPPERCUT"
## EXTENSION THROUGH CLEAN & SNATCH

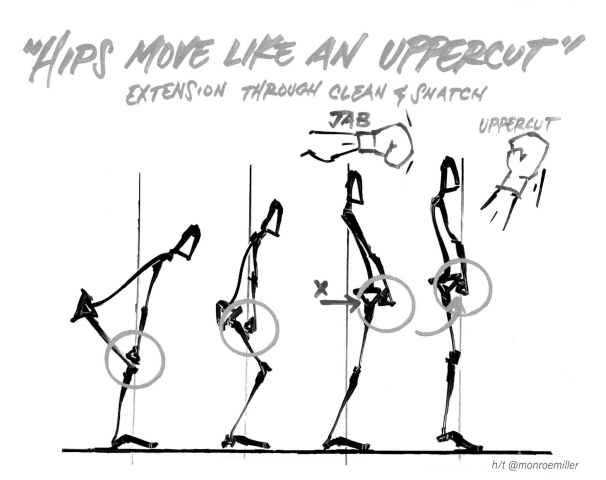

JAB

UPPERCUT

*h/t @monroemiller*

## When?

Extension through the second pull of the clean or snatch

## What does this mean?

During a properly executed clean or snatch, the bar makes contact with the hips. A common mistake that beginners make is thinking they need to smack the bar off their hips during the extension of the second pull.

Rather than "jabbing" your hips forward, the movement of your hips should resemble an "uppercut," driving forward and up.

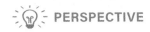

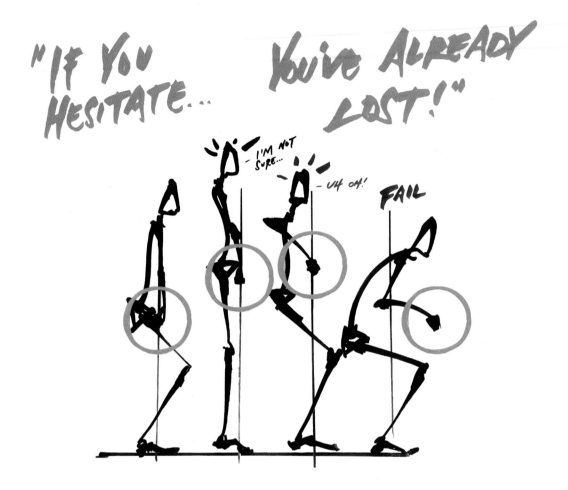

## When?

Clean and snatch

## What does this mean?

When you hesitate, the bar is likely to slow down. If it slows down, it has already won.

## Why is this important?

As a coach, I'd much rather focus on the positive and what the athlete *should* do than what they should *not* do. However, this phrase can be a helpful reminder of the importance of being confident and aggressive when Olympic weightlifting.

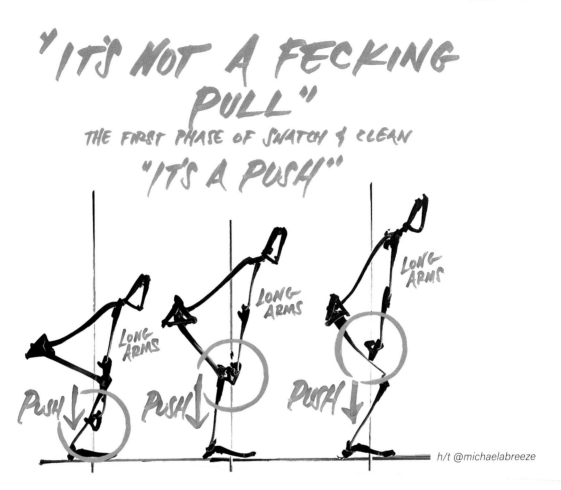

"IT'S NOT A FECKING PULL"

THE FIRST PHASE OF SNATCH & CLEAN

"IT'S A PUSH"

LONG ARMS
LONG ARMS
LONG ARMS
PUSH
PUSH
PUSH

h/t @michaelabreeze

## When?

The first phase of the clean or snatch: floor to above the knee

## What does this mean?

A common descriptor of the initial phase of the clean or snatch is the "first pull." Unfortunately, pulling is an action done with flexion of the shoulder and elbow, neither of which should be moving during this initial phase.

Instead, this phase is more appropriately explained as a leg drive and a push of the feet into the ground.

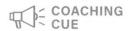
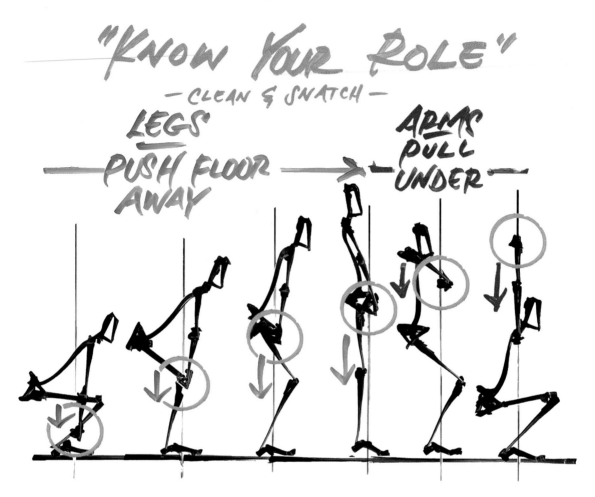

"KNOW YOUR ROLE"
— CLEAN & SNATCH —
LEGS PUSH FLOOR AWAY → ARMS PULL UNDER

## When?

Clean and snatch

## What does this mean?

To simplify the mechanics of the clean and snatch, understand that your legs and arms have two distinctively separate jobs:

- **Legs:** Push the floor away (Phase 1)
- **Arms:** Pull the body under (Phase 2)

# "LEGS DRIVE =THROUGH THE TOES"⇒
## DURING 2ND PULL

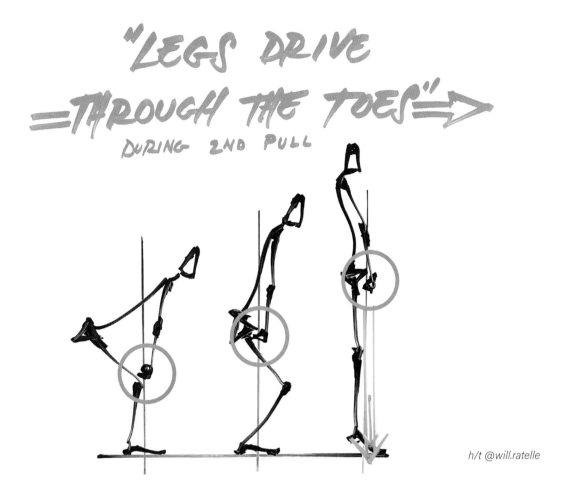

*h/t @will.ratelle*

## When?

Finishing the second pull of the clean and snatch

## What does this mean?

During the hip and knee extension of the second pull, finish the drive through the toes. Imagine the power that you've generated driving through your hips and knees into your toes and against the ground.

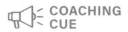
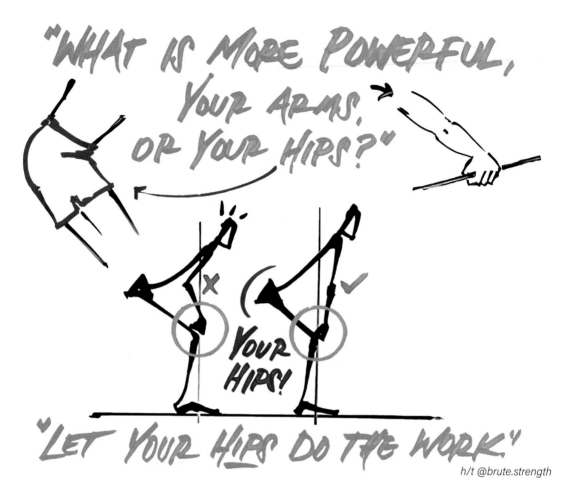

*h/t @brute.strength*

## When?

Addressing early arm bend during the first phase of the snatch and clean

## What does this mean?

When I'm working with a novice lifter and they demonstrate a prominent arm bend during the first phase of the snatch and clean, I say, "What is more powerful: your arms or your hips? Your hips. So let your hips do the work!"

## Why is this important?

When you bend your elbows, the bar loses momentum, which you want to avoid.

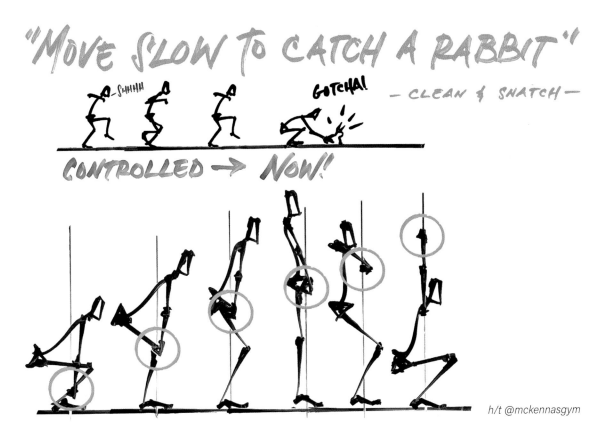

*"MOVE SLOW TO CATCH A RABBIT"*

— CLEAN & SNATCH —

-SHHH!  GOTCHA!

CONTROLLED → NOW!

*h/t @mckennasgym*

## When?

Snatch and clean

## What does this mean?

If you try to sprint after a rabbit, it will simply run away faster than you run, making it impossible to catch. However, if you sneak up on it slowly and time it just right—"GOTCHA!"—you'll be able to catch it.

Similarly, if you immediately jerk the bar off the ground during the snatch or clean, you'll likely miss the proper positioning needed to keep the bar close and receive it.

Start the first pull off the ground smooth and controlled. The bar speed should build as it moves up.

## Why is this important?

Building speed through the first and second pulls allows the lifter to place the bar at the highest position at the right time: the initiation of the third pull.

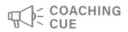
# "MOVE YOUR BODY AROUND THE BAR"

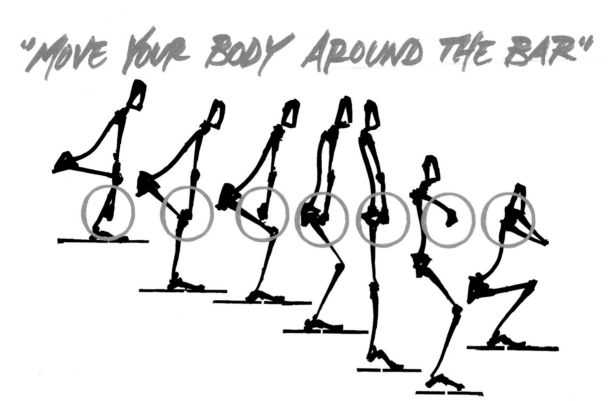

## When?

Clean and snatch

## What does this mean?

Rather than having the bar traveling around the angles of your body (knees and hips), you should aim to keep the bar moving vertically in a straight line and move your body around the bar.

What does it take to move your body around the bar?

- Practice
- Mobility
- Body awareness

## Why is this important?

The objective of Olympic weightlifting is to move the bar vertically (ground to shoulder or overhead) as efficiently as possible. The shortest distance between two points (Point A: ground to Point B: shoulder or overhead) is a straight line.

*Note:* Although the shortest distance between two points is a straight line, the most EFFICIENT bar path for an athlete may not be completely straight.

# "PANDA PULL"

## AKA: CHINESE SNATCH PULL, SNARCH PULL-DOWN

Also known as Chinese snatch pull, snatch fast pull, snatch pull-down, panda snatch pull

## Points of Performance

### Setup:

- Hip-width stance
- Hands on the bar with overhead squat width and a hook grip
- Shoulders slightly in front of bar

### Movement:

- Maintain the lumbar curve.
- Raise your hips and shoulders at the same rate and then extend your hips rapidly.
- Drive your elbows high and to the sides as you move down by bending your hips and knees.
- Keep the bar in immediate proximity to your body.
- As soon as you pull the bar as high as possible, lower it.
- Receive the bar in a power position and then reset.

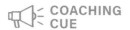
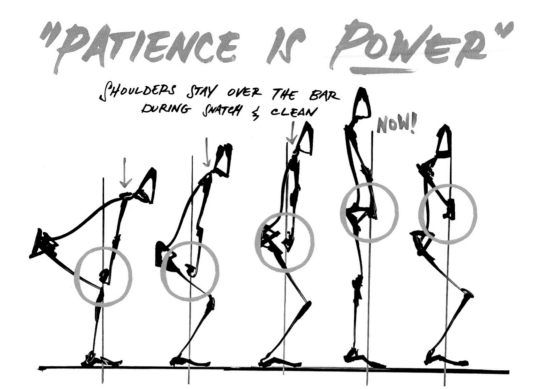

## When?

During the second pull of the clean and snatch

## What does this mean?

During the second pull of the clean and snatch, your knees and hips extend as the bar travels up your thigh.

The longer your shoulders remain over the bar during this extension, the more power you can push into the ground.

Reaching this position requires patience. The more patience you have, the more power you can use.

# "PULL THE BAR APART"

### RECEIVE ON SNATCH

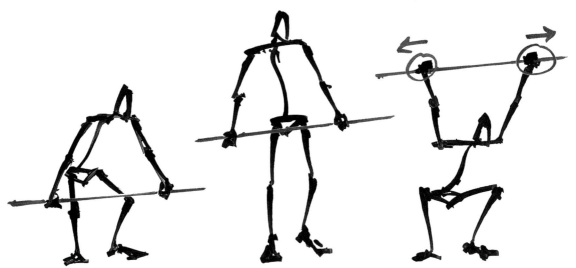

*h/t @k_mighty via @caraheadsslaughter_oly*

## When?

Snatch

## What does this mean?

To create a strong connection with the bar throughout the pull and receive of the snatch, try pulling the bar apart from the center by establishing a strong grip on the bar and pulling toward each end of the bar.

## Why is this important?

This technique engages your shoulders and lats and creates a connection to your body. You're doing more than just holding on to the bar.

As with all cues, give this a try with very light weight and find out if it makes a difference for you.

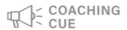
# "PULL UP YOUR SWEATPANTS"

## CLEAN HIGH PULL

ELBOWS DRIVE
HIGH & BACK

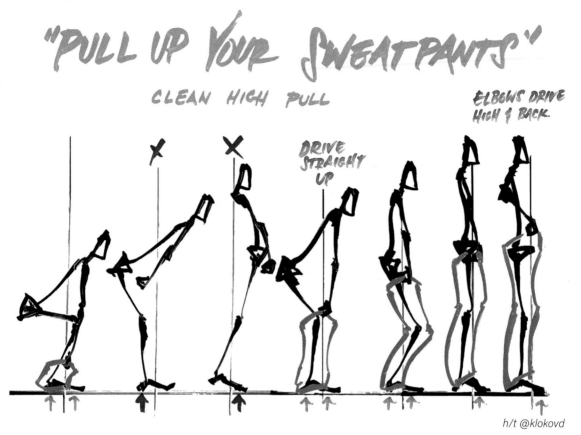

DRIVE
STRAIGHT
UP

*h/t @klokovd*

## When?

Clean high pull

## What does this mean?

The clean high pull and pulling up your sweatpants are the same movement. Stay balanced through the whole foot as you drive your feet into the ground and stand up. Keep the bar path vertical, as if you're pulling up your sweatpants.

## Why is this important?

A common error with the clean pull is driving too hard through the heels and then heavily shifting balance to the toes during extension of the knees and hips. The result is the bar path looping back and forward.

# "PULL YOURSELF UNDER THE BAR."

## CLEAN & SNATCH THIRD PULL

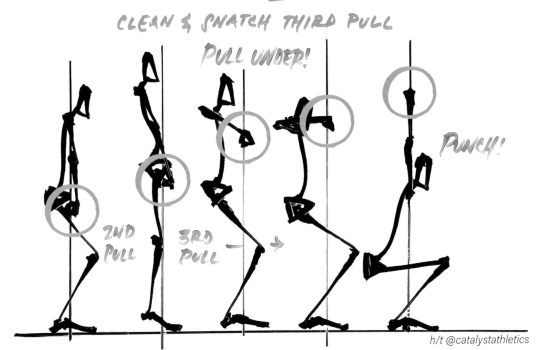

PULL UNDER!

2ND PULL

3RD PULL

PUNCH!

*h/t @catalystathletics*

### When?
During the third pull of the clean or snatch

### What does this mean?
Immediately after you extend your hips and knees, you must continue to keep tension on the bar and pull yourself *under* the bar into the receiving position.

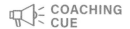
# "RELEASE THE HOOK GRIP"
## - DURING THE CLEAN RECEIVE -

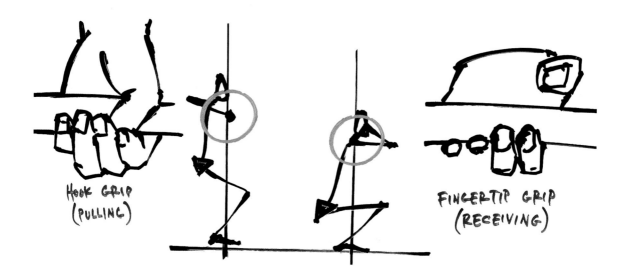

HOOK GRIP
(PULLING)

FINGERTIP GRIP
(RECEIVING)

### When?

Receiving the bar during the clean turnover

### What does this mean?

A common error that I see with beginning Olympic lifters is receiving the bar with "slow and low" elbows during the clean turnover. Many times, the cause of this is that the lifter is keeping a firm hook grip on the bar after their elbows have passed in front of the bar. Instead, they should release the hook grip on the bar and switch to a fingertip grip.

### Why is this important?

Releasing the hook grip on the bar but keeping the bar within the fingers during the clean turnover places you in a better position to get your elbows higher quickly.

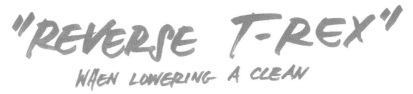

# "REVERSE T-REX"
## WHEN LOWERING A CLEAN

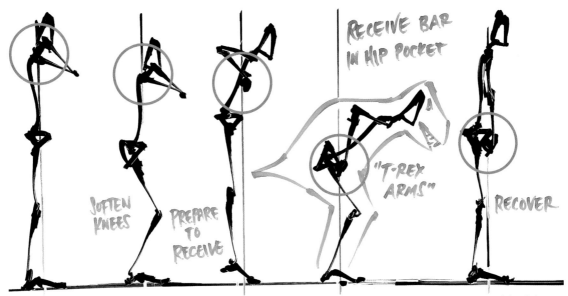

RECEIVE BAR IN HIP POCKET

"T-REX ARMS"

SOFTEN KNEES

PREPARE TO RECEIVE

RECOVER

*h/t @michaelabreeze*

## When?

Lowering the clean

## What does this mean?

When you're lowering the bar from the front-rack position, bring your elbows back and allow the bar to drop. Keep the bar as close to your torso as possible and receive the bar in your hip pocket with your bum back, arms bent, and soft knees. This position loosely resembles a Tyrannosaurus rex.

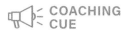
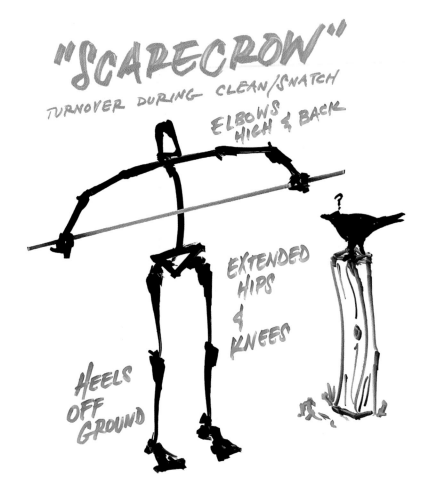

"SCARECROW"
TURNOVER DURING CLEAN/SNATCH
ELBOWS HIGH & BACK
EXTENDED HIPS & KNEES
HEELS OFF GROUND

## When?

Body position when describing turnover during the snatch or clean

## What does this mean?

The "scarecrow" position occurs when you reach extension through your hips and knees with your heels off the ground, elbows at shoulder height, and bar close to your chest.

## Why is this important?

Since the turnover can be especially tricky for beginners, pausing at this position with very light weight may help you build body awareness.

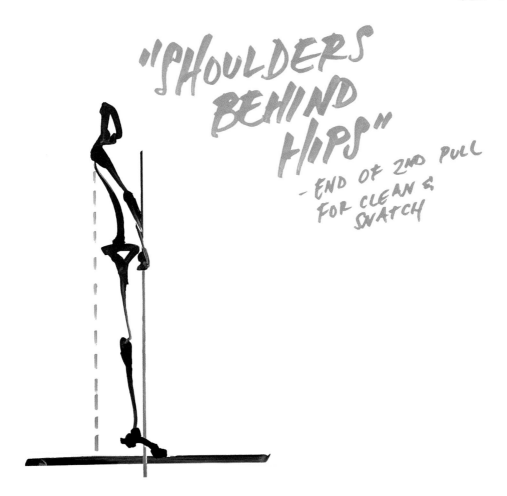

"SHOULDERS BEHIND HIPS"

- END OF 2ND PULL FOR CLEAN & SNATCH

### When?

Describing the end of the second pull

### What does this mean?

In the final position of the second pull, your legs will be vertically extended, and your shoulders will be behind your hips.

### Why is this important?

This position allows the bar to continue its vertical trajectory.

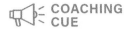

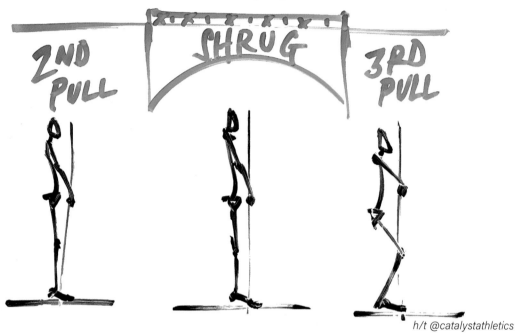

*h/t @catalystathletics*

## When?

During clean or snatch

## What does this mean?

At the end of the second pull, the shrug initiates the third pull—the pull under the bar. Your arms don't bend until after the shrug.

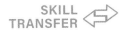
# SKILL TRANSFER
## BOX JUMPS → HANG CLEANS

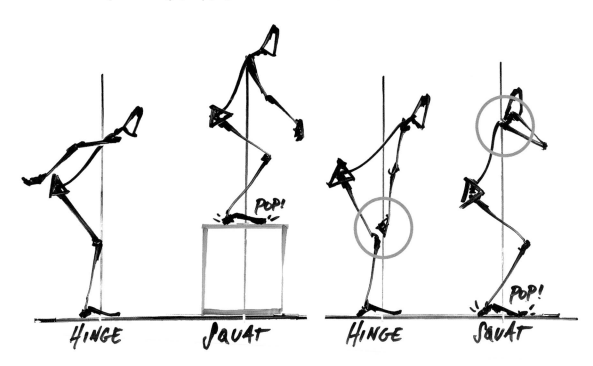

HINGE          SQUAT          HINGE          SQUAT

**Jump and land in box jumps —> Hang clean start and receive**

Both of these movements start in a hinge and finish in a squat. In addition, sticking the landing during a box jump is akin to receiving the bar with flat feet.

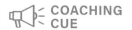
## COACHING CUE

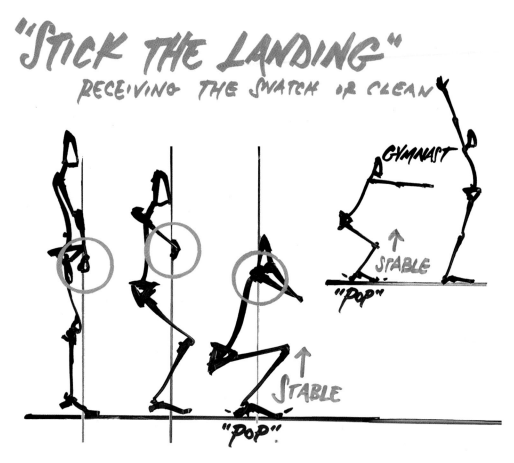

"STICK THE LANDING"
RECEIVING THE SNATCH OR CLEAN

GYMNAST
↑ STABLE
"POP"
↑ STABLE
"POP"

## When?

Receiving the clean or snatch

## What does this mean?

When you receive the bar, demonstrate body control and careful positioning as if you're a gymnast landing a dismount. After extending through the hip and knees during the second pull, you need to reposition your feet to the receiving stance. The reconnection of your feet to the floor should be fast and aggressive. Both feet should make immediate full contact with the floor to create a stable connection from the ground up.

# "THE TEN CLEAN COMMANDMENTS"

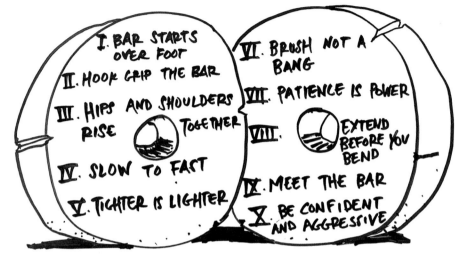

I. BAR STARTS OVER FOOT
II. HOOK GRIP THE BAR
III. HIPS AND SHOULDERS RISE TOGETHER
IV. SLOW TO FAST
V. TIGHTER IS LIGHTER
VI. BRUSH NOT A BANG
VII. PATIENCE IS POWER
VIII. EXTEND BEFORE YOU BEND
IX. MEET THE BAR
X. BE CONFIDENT AND AGGRESSIVE

## When?

Cleans and snatches

## What does this mean?

**Here are "The Ten Clean (and Snatch) Commandments":**

1. **Bar starts over the foot:** The exact location varies based on your limb length.

2. **Hook grip the bar:** The hook grip is an eventual necessity if you want to increase the weight you can clean and snatch.

3. **Hips and shoulders rise together:** To apply even pressure into the ground and set your body in the optimal position for the second pull, your hips and shoulders should rise at the same rate through the first pull.

4. **Slow to fast:** The bar speed increases throughout the first and second pulls with a crescendo at the end of the second pull.

5. **Tighter is lighter:** The farther the weight is from your body, the heavier it will feel.

6. **Brush not a bang:** During the second pull, the bar brushes up your body (your hips for the clean or your upper thighs for the snatch). Your hips should not bang the bar forward.

7. **Patience is power:** The longer your shoulders stay over the bar during the first and second pulls, the more vertical power you can generate.

8. **Extend before you bend:** Your hips should fully extend during the second pull before you bend your knees, hips, and arms during the third pull.

9. **Meet the bar:** You should receive the bar in the front rack at the same moment your feet hit the floor.

10. **Be confident and aggressive:** The Olympic lifts are not for the timid. If you hesitate at all, the bar will win.

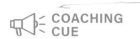

# THE SNATCH & CLEAN ARE TRANSFORMERS.

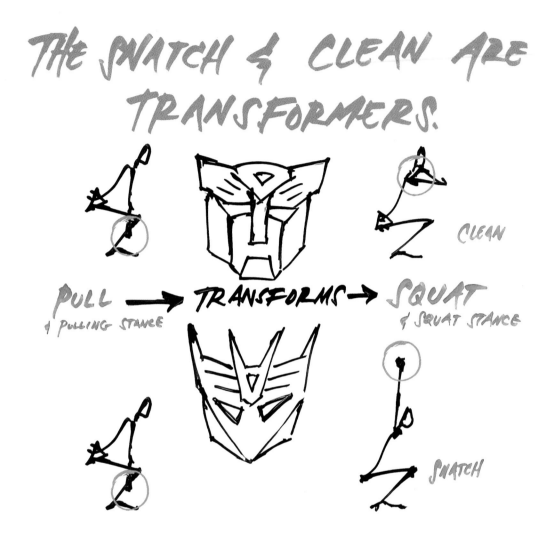

PULL ⟶ TRANSFORMS ⟶ SQUAT
& PULLING STANCE                    & SQUAT STANCE

CLEAN

SNATCH

## When?

Describing the snatch and clean and their stances

## What does this mean?

The snatch and the clean are Transformers. They transform from a pull to a squat (front: clean, overhead: snatch).

In doing so, they must also transform from a pulling stance (approximately hip width) to a squat stance (approximately shoulder width).

# "UP NOT OUT"
### SNATCH & CLEAN BAR PATH

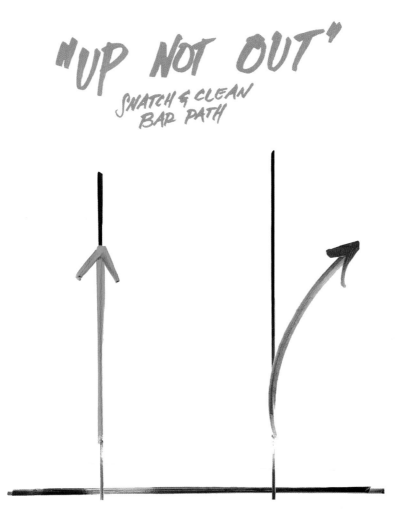

## When?

Describing the bar path for the snatch and the clean

## What does this mean?

There are times when I need to remind my athletes that Olympic weightlifting is a vertical sport. We want to do all we can to move the bar *up*. Yes, there are small deviations in the line of the bar path, but these should not be the focus of concern for the novice lifter.

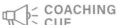
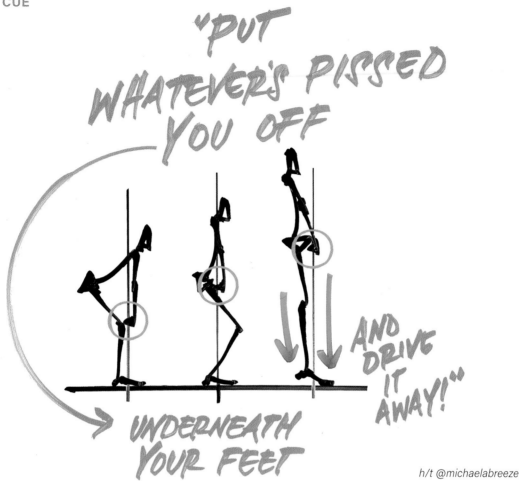

"PUT WHATEVER'S PISSED YOU OFF

UNDERNEATH YOUR FEET

AND DRIVE IT AWAY!"

*h/t @michaelabreeze*

## When?

Extension of knees and hips during the clean or snatch

## What does this mean?

This creative external cue transforms the powerful use of emotions into an aggressive physical action, taking something negative and turning it into something positive.

Furthermore, this idea might help you understand the necessary force to drive into the ground when reaching extension in the clean or snatch.

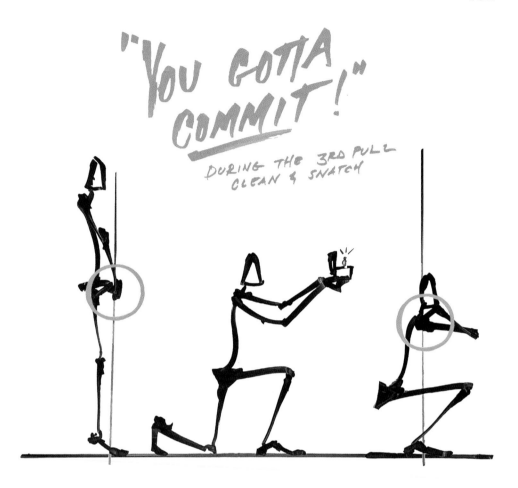

"YOU GOTTA COMMIT!"

DURING THE 3RD PULL
CLEAN & SNATCH

## When?

The third pull of the clean or snatch

## What does this mean?

If you want your relationship with the bar to have a chance at success, you need to commit to pulling yourself under to receive (as you might commit yourself to a relationship).

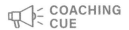 

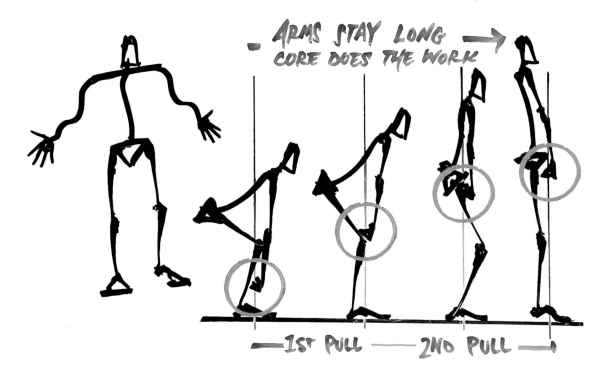

"ARMS ARE ROPES"

DURING 1ST & 2ND PULL OF CLEAN & SNATCH

ARMS STAY LONG →
CORE DOES THE WORK

— 1ST PULL — 2ND PULL —

## When?

First and second pulls of the clean and snatch

## What does this mean?

Before you extend your hips and knees, your arms hang long and relaxed (like ropes) with your hands "attached" to the bar.

## Why is this important?

This technique creates an efficient transfer of power from your core to the bar.

# "CONTROLLED OFF THE FLOOR, HARD AFTER THE KNEES."

### BUILDING BAR SPEED

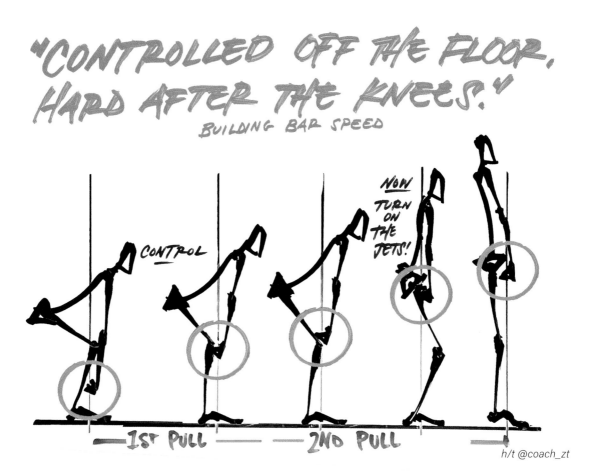

CONTROL

NOW TURN ON THE JETS!

— 1ST PULL — — 2ND PULL —

*h/t @coach_zt*

## When?

Describing bar speed from the floor to extension

## What does this mean?

Building speed through the first and second pulls allows you to place the bar at the highest position at the right time—the initiation of the third pull.

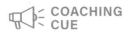
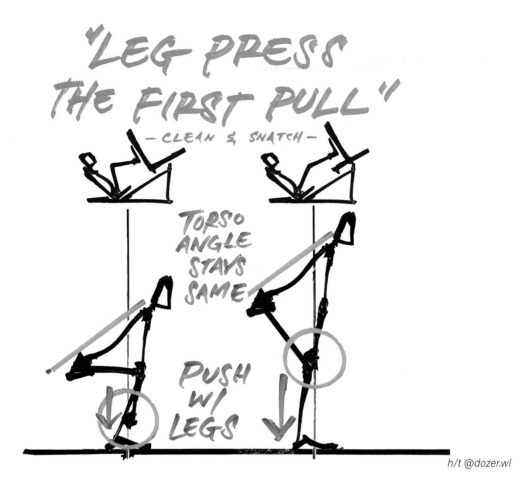

*h/t @dozer.wl*

## When?

Initiating the first pull of the clean or snatch

## What does this mean?

Your hips and shoulders should rise at the same rate during the first pull of the clean or snatch. When you keep them in sync, the angle of your torso stays the same throughout the first pull.

This is accomplished by driving your legs into the ground with even pressure through your feet.

The movement is similar to a seated leg press, where your torso does not change as you push your feet against the weight.

*Note:* This cue has been a game-changer for me. I hope it helps you.

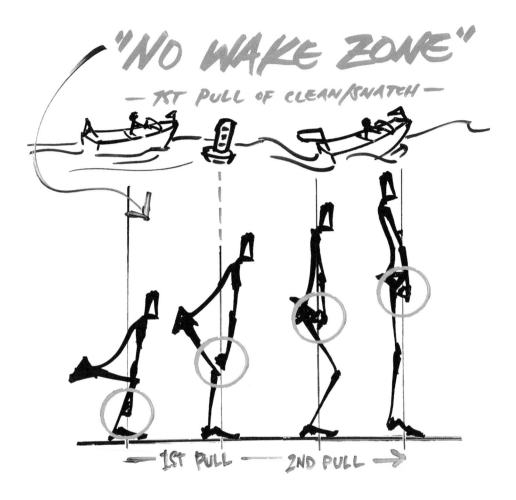

"NO WAKE ZONE"
— 1ST PULL OF CLEAN/SNATCH —

— 1ST PULL — 2ND PULL →

## When?

First pull of the clean or snatch

## What does this mean?

When boating, the no wake zone is an area where boats must travel without creating any waves. Similarly, the first pull of the clean or snatch should be smooth and in control.

Once the lift enters the second pull (the boat leaves the wake zone), the lifter can really lay on the gas!

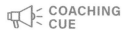

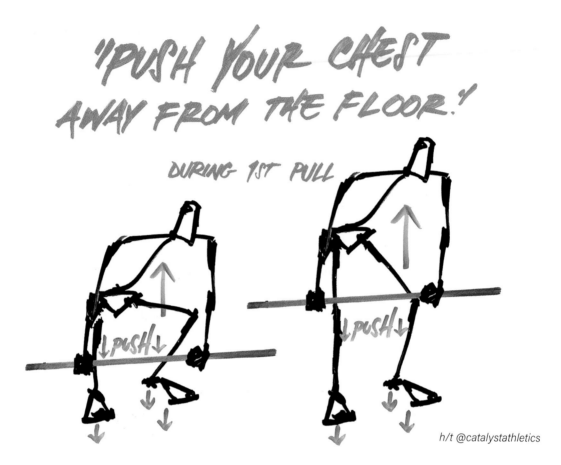

"PUSH YOUR CHEST AWAY FROM THE FLOOR."

DURING 1ST PULL

↓ PUSH ↓

↓ PUSH ↓

*h/t @catalystathletics*

### When?

First pull (floor to above the knee) of the clean or snatch

### What does this mean?

A common error during the first pull is the hips rising faster than the shoulders. This results in a leak of power and places the lifter in a less-optimal position.

Rather than thinking of pulling the bar off the ground, focus more on holding on to the bar and pushing your chest away from the ground.

# "SQUAT THE 1ST PULL"
## — CLEAN & SNATCH —

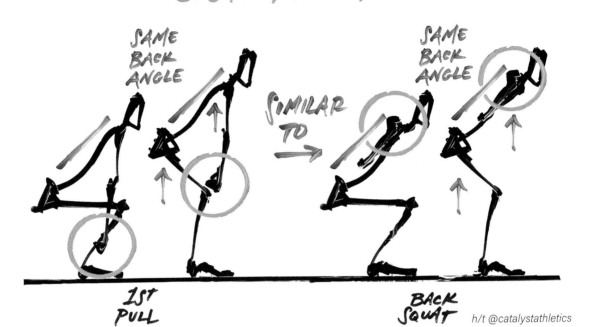

SAME
BACK
ANGLE

SIMILAR
TO

SAME
BACK
ANGLE

1ST
PULL

BACK
SQUAT

*h/t @catalystathletics*

**When?**

First pull of snatch and clean

**What does this mean?**

The first pull should be a squatting motion but without extending your hips. Push through your whole foot and think of moving your body up without changing your back's angle.

**Why is this important?**

Doing the first pull this way helps put you into the optimal position for the second pull.

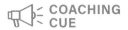

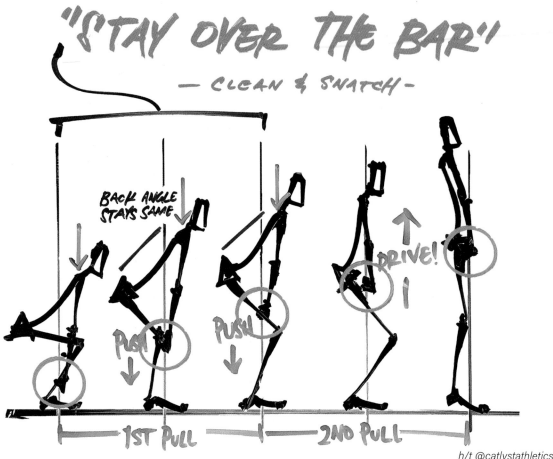

# "STAY OVER THE BAR"
## — CLEAN & SNATCH —

BACK ANGLE STAYS SAME

PUSH

PUSH

DRIVE!

1ST PULL ———— 2ND PULL

*h/t @catlystathletics*

## When?

Body and bar position from the ground to the mid-thigh during the clean and snatch

## What does this mean?

Stay over the bar by pushing with your legs and maintaining the same back angle until you initiate the second pull at your thigh.

## Why is this important?

Your shoulders do and must move behind the bar at the end of the (second) pull of a clean or snatch. This technique helps you keep your shoulders behind the bar.

# "BAR BRUSHES BELT BUCKLE"
## — KEEP BAR CLOSE DURING SECOND PULL —

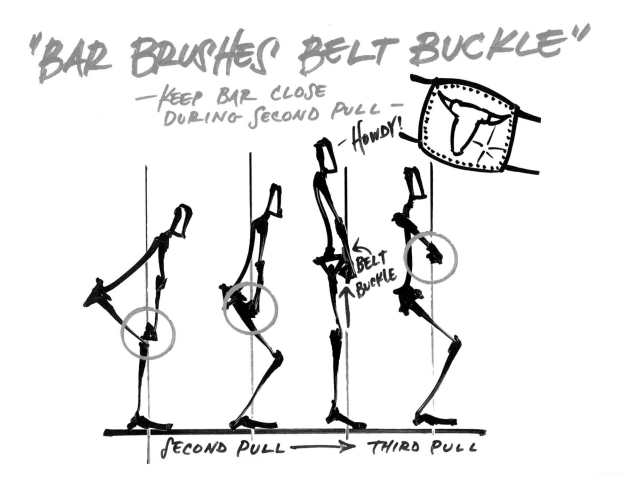

— HOWDY!

BELT BUCKLE

SECOND PULL ——> THIRD PULL

## When?

For hitting/brushing the hip pocket during the clean and snatch

## What does this mean?

During the second pull of the clean and snatch, the bar needs to be as close to your body as possible without dragging. As the bar passes your hips, imagine it's brushing against your belt buckle.

*Note:* For more information, please read "Hips, Meet Bar: Bar-Body Contact in the Extension of the Snatch and Clean" on the Catalyst Athletics website.

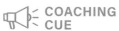

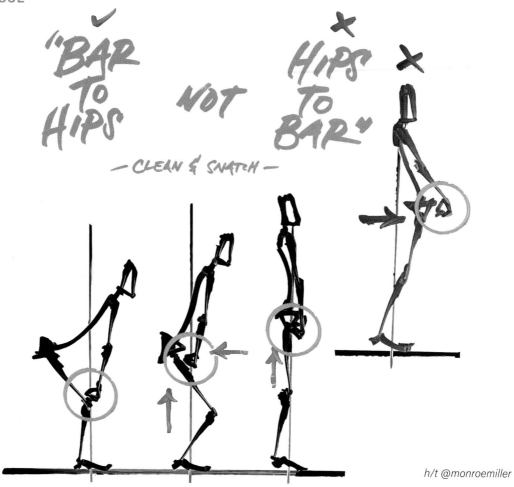

"BAR TO HIPS" ✔ NOT HIPS TO BAR ✗

— CLEAN & SNATCH —

*h/t @monroemiller*

## When?

Describing hip contact with the bar during extension of the clean or snatch

## What does this mean?

During the second pull of the clean and snatch, the bar makes contact with your body (your upper thigh for the clean or your hips during the snatch).

Focusing on keeping the bar close to your body as you extend your hips and knees keeps the bar path moving vertically.

# EXTENSION = DENTIST'S OFFICE
## - CLEAN & SNATCH -

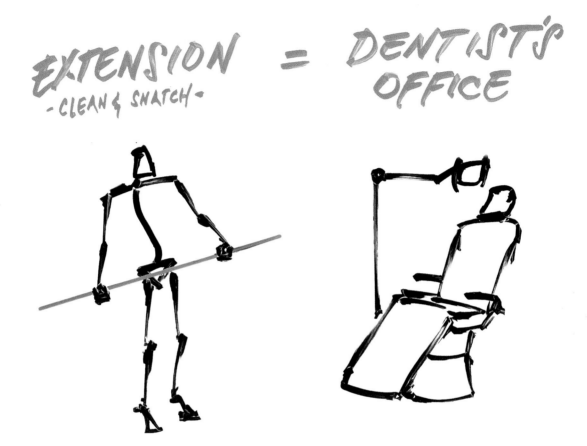

## When?

Clean and snatch

## What does this mean?

Extension is someplace you *must* go (just like you must go to the dentist's office), but you want to spend as little time there as possible.

To receive the bar in a strong and stable position, your hips must flex just as aggressively as they extended during the second pull. Hit extension and then immediately flex your hips and knees.

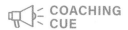
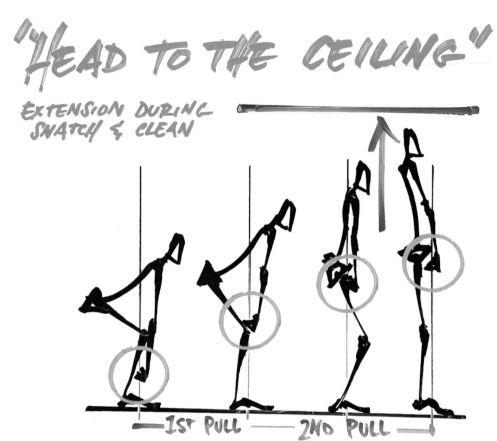

*"HEAD TO THE CEILING"*

EXTENSION DURING
SNATCH & CLEAN

1ST PULL ——— 2ND PULL

## When?

Extension during the snatch or clean

## What does this mean?

In an effort to reach maximum power during the second pull, you should reach full extension through your hips and knees, similar to the way you jump.

The idea of driving your head to the ceiling may be a relatable movement pattern that helps you target this extension.

# "THE LAUNCH POINT"
## THE POWER POSITION
## CLEAN & SNATCH

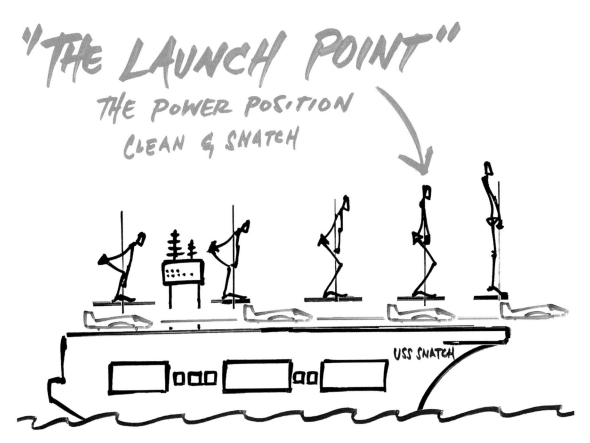

USS SNATCH

## What does this mean?

The launch point is the power position of the clean and the snatch. It occurs at the end of the scoop, the point at which your knees are the farthest forward at the top of the pull.

Your trunk is approximately vertical, and the bar is at its final full contact with your body (i.e., your hips during the snatch and your upper thighs and hips for the clean).

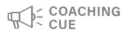
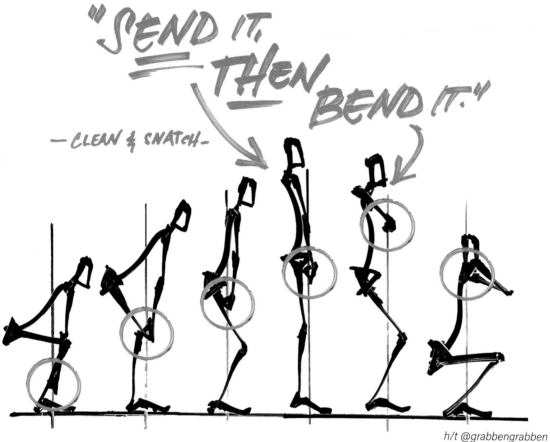

"SEND IT, THEN BEND IT."

— CLEAN & SNATCH —

*h/t @grabbengrabben*

## When?

Clean and snatch

## What does this mean?

**Send it:** Keep your arms long and aggressively extend your hips and knees during the final upward explosion of the second pull.

THEN

**Bend it:** Bend your elbows and legs to pull under the bar to receive.

*— CLEAN/SNATCH —*

# "ONCE THE BAR PASSES THE KNEES... *SEND IT!!*"

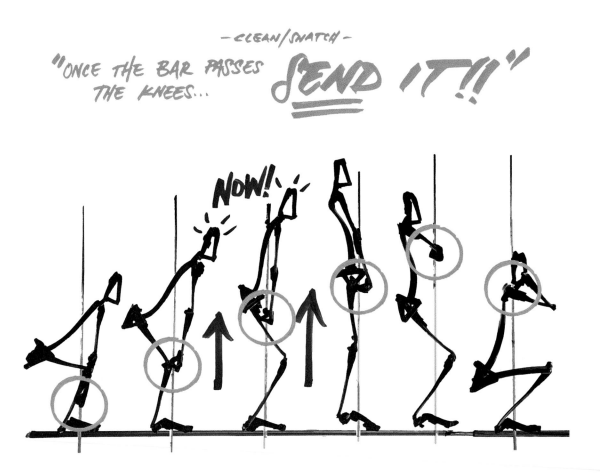

NOW!

## When?

Clean and snatch

## What does this mean?

When working with novice lifters, I've noticed the "complexity" of the third pull and receive can be a source uncertainty—to the point the lifter hesitates through the second pull. If the lifter hesitates, the bar speed stops. The extension of the second pull *must* be explosive, and the lifter must be aggressive. They need to *send it*!

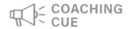 

# "TRIGGER AT YOUR HIPS"
## —SNATCH—
### "TRIGGER AT YOUR UPPER THIGH" —FOR CLEAN

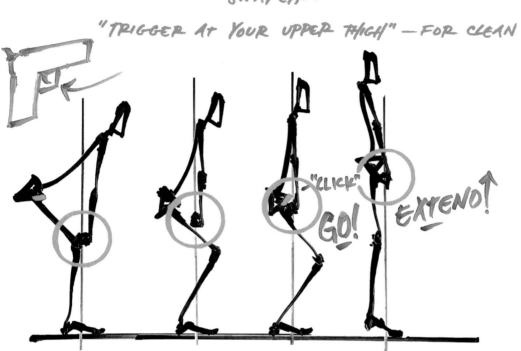

## When?

Snatch (or trigger at your upper thigh for the clean)

## What does this mean?

During the second pull of the clean and snatch, your knees and hips extend as the bar travels up the thigh.

Consequently, you can imagine there is a trigger at your hips during the snatch (or your upper thigh for a clean). Once the bar touches the trigger (not before), you've received the sign to finish your hip extension violently and aggressively.

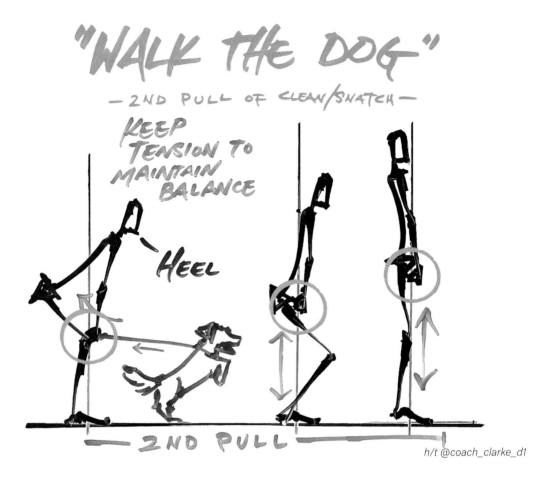

"WALK THE DOG"

— 2ND PULL OF CLEAN/SNATCH —

KEEP
TENSION TO
MAINTAIN
BALANCE

HEEL

— 2ND PULL —

h/t @coach_clarke_d1

## When?

Second pull of the clean or snatch

## What does this mean?

Throughout the second pull of the clean and snatch, maintain the balance of the bar/body system over your feet and keep the bar as close to your body as possible through the upward drive. This is similar to keeping the tension on the leash of an excited dog.

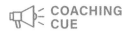
# BAR = AXLE
# ELBOWS = WHEEL
## DURING CLEAN RECEIVE

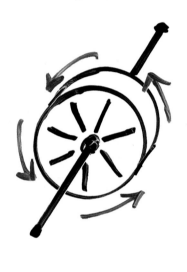

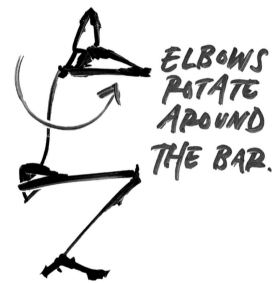

ELBOWS
ROTATE
AROUND
THE BAR.

### When?
Receiving the bar during the clean

### What does this mean?
In this analogy, the bar is the center axis as your elbows rotate around to the front-rack position.

### Why is this important?
Describing the receive this way may help lifters understand its mechanics.

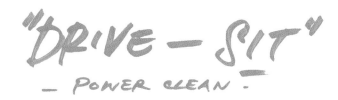

## "DRIVE — SIT"
### — POWER CLEAN —

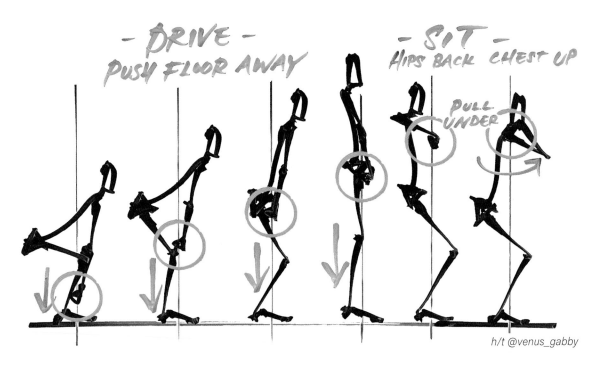

**— DRIVE —**
**PUSH FLOOR AWAY**

**— SIT —**
**HIPS BACK CHEST UP**

**PULL UNDER**

h/t @venus_gabby

## When?

Power clean

## What does this mean?

**Drive:** During the first and second pulls of the power clean, drive the bar up by pushing the floor away.

**Sit:** Immediately upon reaching extension through your hips and knees, use your arms to pull your body under the bar, receiving the bar with your hips, back, and chest up, as if you are taking a seat in a chair.

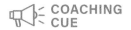
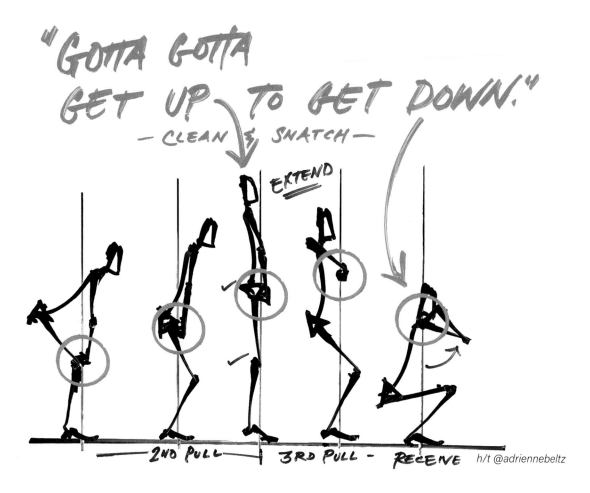

"GOTTA GOTTA GET UP TO GET DOWN."
— CLEAN & SNATCH —

EXTEND

2ND PULL — 3RD PULL - RECEIVE

*h/t @adriennebeltz*

## When?

Extension during the snatch or clean

## What does this mean?

In an effort to reach maximum power during the second pull, you should reach full extension through your hips and knees.

## Why is this important?

Thinking about getting *all* the way *up* before you pull down under the bar may be a relatable concept that helps you target this extension.

# "TAKE A SEAT"
## DURING POWER CLEAN

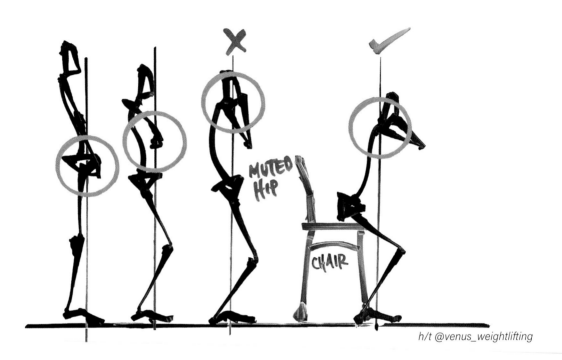

h/t @venus_weightlifting

## When?

Power clean

## What does this mean?

A common error during the power clean, especially for novice lifters, is receiving the bar with muted hip function. This posture results from the legs compensating for the hips' failure to flex.

To combat this, focus on receiving the bar with your hips back and chest up, as if you're taking a seat in a chair.

## Why is this important?

This balanced position provides a more stable and efficient movement pattern, especially as the weight gets heavier.

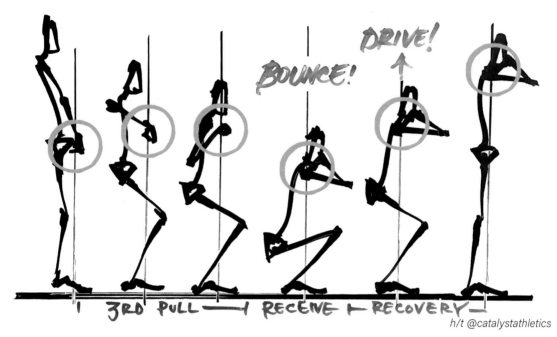

"THE BOUNCE"
DRIVING UP FROM CLEAN/SQUAT

BOUNCE!

DRIVE!

| 3RD PULL | RECEIVE | RECOVERY |

*h/t @catalystathletics*

## What does this mean?

The bounce refers to the elastic rebound at the bottom of the squat or the clean, which allows for easier and quicker recovery from the bottom position.

When you do the bounce, you coordinate the upward bounce of your upper leg off your lower leg, the stretch shortening reflex in your leg and hip muscles, and the whip of the bar.

Check out "Learn & Train the Bounce in the Clean for Better Recoveries."

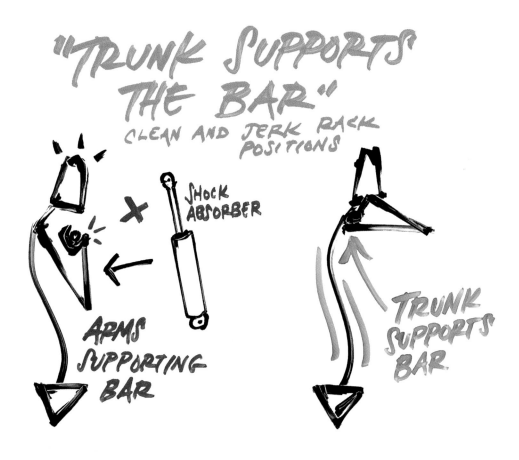

"TRUNK SUPPORTS THE BAR"

CLEAN AND JERK RACK POSITIONS

SHOCK ABSORBER

ARMS SUPPORTING BAR

TRUNK SUPPORTS BAR

## When?

Clean rack and jerk rack positions

## What does this mean?

The primary similarity between the clean rack position (as in the front squat) and the jerk rack position is that the bar is directly supported by the trunk.

## Why is this important?

A secure connection must be made between your trunk and the barbell to stabilize the bar and create an efficient transfer of power from your lower body.

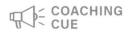

**COACHING CUE**

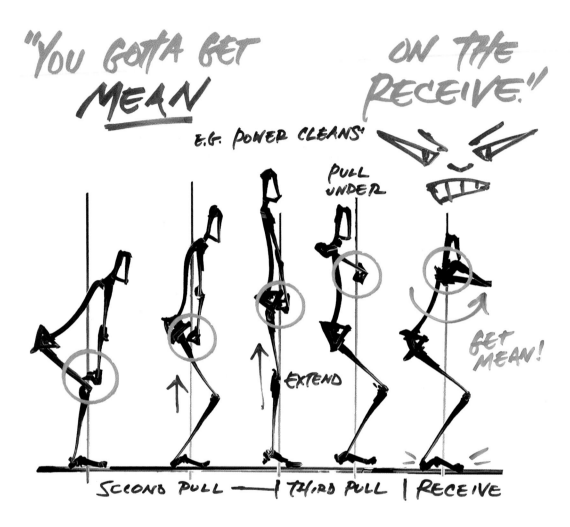

"YOU GOTTA GET **MEAN** ON THE RECEIVE."

E.G. POWER CLEANS!

PULL UNDER

EXTEND

GET MEAN!

SECOND PULL — | THIRD PULL | RECEIVE

**When?**

Clean and snatch

**What does this mean?**

The receive of the clean and snatch *must* be aggressive.

**Why is this important?**

The clean and snatch are typically executed in single or small repetitions and with heavy weight (relative to your strength). When operating with heavy weight, you must assert full and complete effort, or "the bar will win."

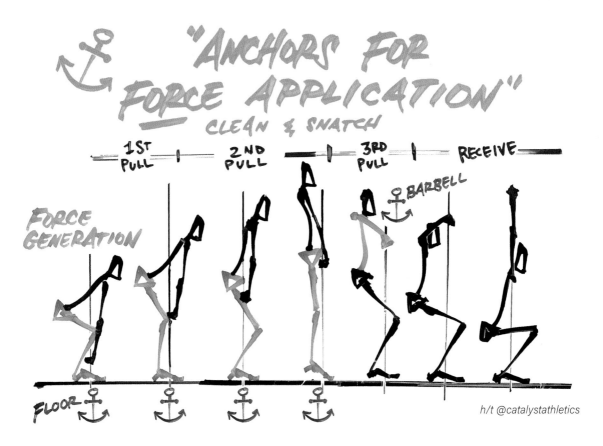

## "ANCHORS FOR FORCE APPLICATION"
### CLEAN & SNATCH

1ST PULL — 2ND PULL — 3RD PULL — RECEIVE

FORCE GENERATION

BARBELL

FLOOR

*h/t @catalystathletics*

### When?

Clean and snatch

### What does this mean?

An anchor of force application is the location that receives the generated force. During the first and second pulls of the clean and snatch, you engage your core and generate force with your lower body, using the ground as the anchor for force application.

During the third pull, you generate force with your upper body and pull under the barbell, using the barbell as the anchor of force application.

### Why is this important?

During a complex movement like the clean and snatch, it's important to know what parts of your body are responsible for creating force and when they're doing it. It's similar to an orchestra playing a symphony; the tuba section needs to wait for the clarinets to create a harmonious performance.

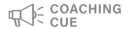
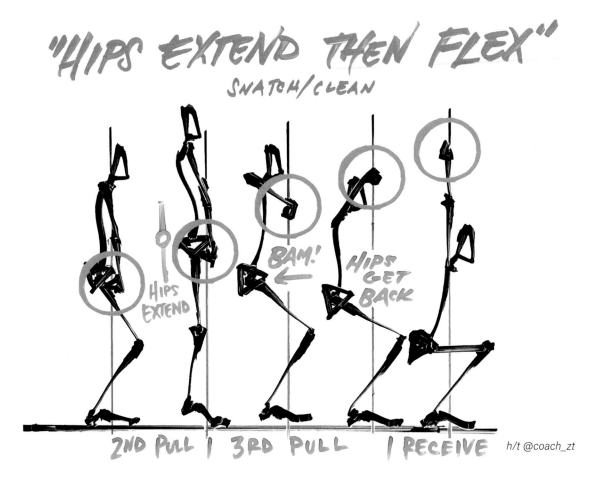

# "HIPS EXTEND THEN FLEX"
## SNATCH/CLEAN

HIPS EXTEND

BAM!

HIPS GET BACK

2ND PULL | 3RD PULL | RECEIVE

*h/t @coach_zt*

## When?

The transition from the second pull to the third pull of the snatch and clean

## What does this mean?

Much of the focus with the clean and snatch is explosive hip extension. This is vital to the vertical propulsion of the bar. However, in an effort to receive the bar in a strong and stable position, your hips must flex just as aggressively as they extended during the second pull.

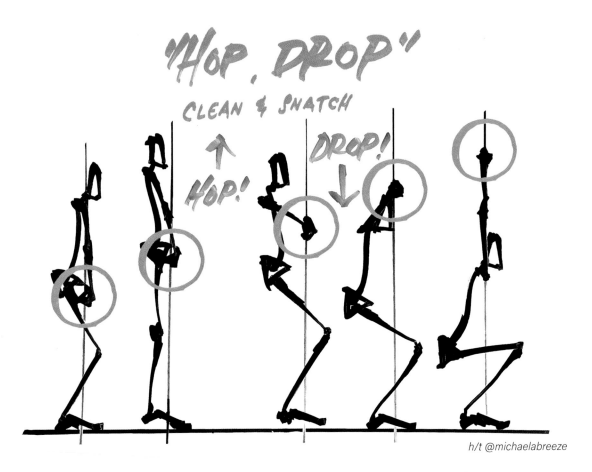

"HOP, DROP"
CLEAN & SNATCH
↑
HOP!
DROP!
↓

*h/t @michaelabreeze*

## When?

Snatch and clean

## What does this mean?

A common error during extension is the lifter throwing their head and shoulders backward and driving their hips forward, which also sends the bar forward. To stay balanced in this situation, the lifter must then whip the bar back toward the midline.

Instead, the movement of your hips should be vertical, similar to a hop. Then you immediately drop down into the receive position.

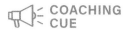
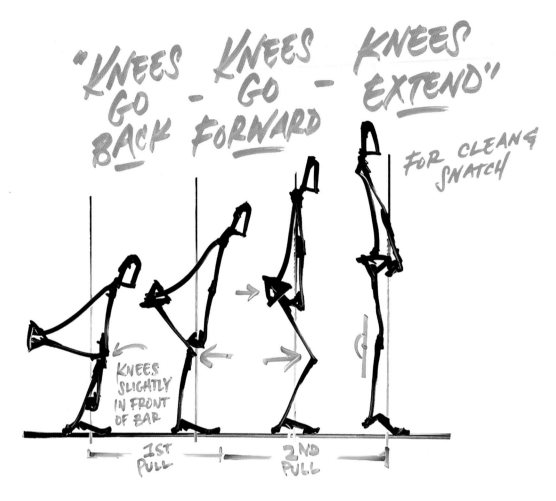

"KNEES GO BACK - KNEES GO FORWARD - KNEES EXTEND"

FOR CLEAN & SNATCH

KNEES SLIGHTLY IN FRONT OF BAR

1ST PULL

2ND PULL

## When?

Describing the first and second pulls of the clean or snatch

## What does this mean?

In the setup of the clean or snatch, your knees are slightly in front of the bar. During the first pull, your back angle stays relatively the same, and your knees move behind the bar to allow the bar to travel in a relatively straight line from the floor to above the knee.

At the initiation of the second pull, your knees move forward of the bar as your body repositions to allow the application of vertical force. As you continue to drive through the legs, the second pull finishes with your knees and hips extending.

# "PUSH BEFORE YOU PULL"
## — SNATCH & CLEAN —

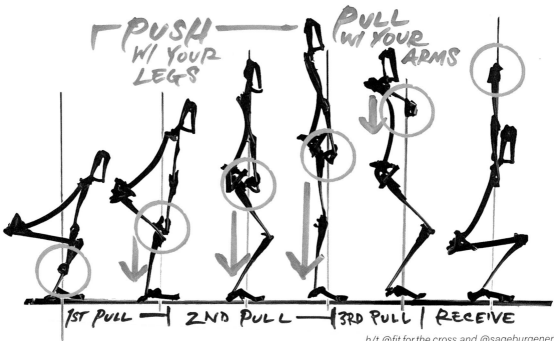

PUSH W/ YOUR LEGS

PULL W/ YOUR ARMS

1ST PULL — 2ND PULL — 3RD PULL | RECEIVE

*h/t @fit.for.the.cross and @sageburgener*

## When?

Sequence for snatch and clean

## What does this mean?

Push with your legs before you pull under the bar.

During the first and second pulls of the snatch, focus on pushing with your legs against the ground. Upon reaching full extension through your hips and knees, pull yourself under the bar.

## Why is this important?

This cue is a reminder not to bend your arms early before you've reached full extension with your hips and knees.

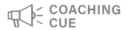

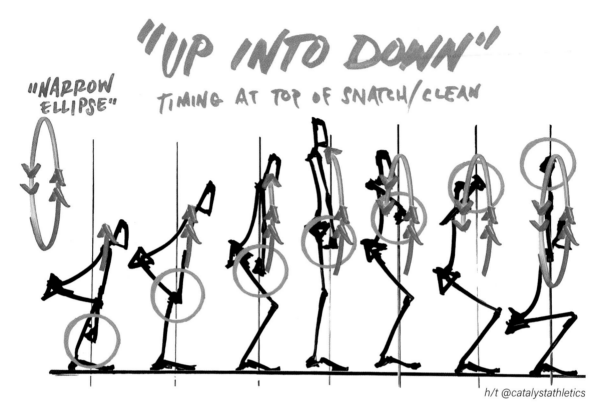

"NARROW ELLIPSE"

"UP INTO DOWN"

TIMING AT TOP OF SNATCH/CLEAN

*h/t @catalystathletics*

## When?

Timing at the top of the pull for the clean and snatch

## What does this mean?

The focus for teaching the movement progressions of the clean and snatch is commonly on the segments of the overall pattern:

- The second pull and then the receive

- The extension and then the flexion

The idea of separate segments might inadvertently cause the lifter to delay the transition between the top of the pull and receiving the bar in the rack position. What you really want in the execution is a fluid, continuous, uninterrupted motion. Think of the transition as up into down, similar to the motion you'd make to create a narrow ellipse.

# "HUMAN VERSION OF A SQUAT RACK"

## – SNATCH RECEIVE –

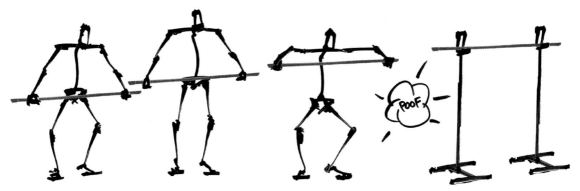

h/t @venus_gabby

## When?

Snatch receive

## What does this mean?

As the bar continues its upward drive at the end of the second pull of the snatch, you must immediately and aggressively pull under to receive the bar in a strong and stable position, as if you are a human squat rack. Your mid-foot, shoulders, and the bar should be in a straight line to create balance as you stabilize and stand.

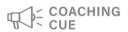
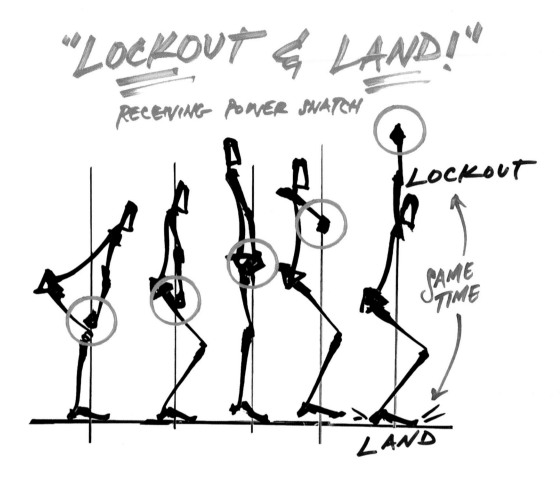

## When?

Timing the receive of the power snatch

## What does this mean?

When receiving the bar during the power snatch, you should aggressively punch the bar overhead. The lockout from this punch should happen at the same time you reconnect your feet to the floor (in other words, at the same time you land).

A sharp "pop" of your feet against the floor indicates you have aggressively reconnected and are stable from the ground up.

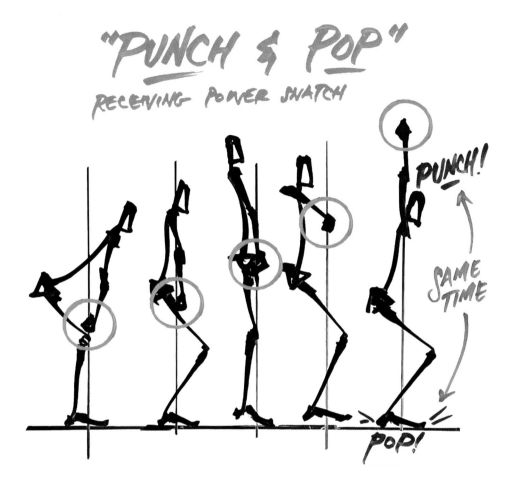

"PUNCH & POP"
RECEIVING POWER SNATCH

PUNCH!
SAME TIME
POP!

## When?

Timing the receive of the power snatch

## What does this mean?

When receiving the bar during the power snatch, you should aggressively punch the bar overhead. The lockout from this punch should happen at the same time you reconnect your feet to the floor.

A sharp "pop" of your feet against the floor indicates you have aggressively reconnected and are stable from the ground up.

# "STICK - STABILIZE - STAND"
## RECEIVING THE SNATCH

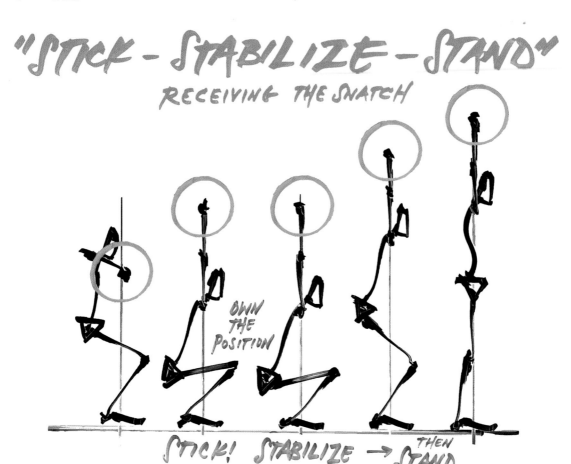

OWN THE POSITION

STICK! STABILIZE → THEN STAND

## When?

Receiving the snatch

## What does this mean?

**Stick:** Similar to a gymnast, you need to stick the landing for a snatch. After extending through your hips and knees during the second pull, you need to reposition your feet to the receiving stance. Both feet should make immediate full contact with the floor to create a stable connection from the ground up.

**Stabilize:** Take a moment to "own your position" to

- Build body and spatial awareness
- Build body control
- Build self-confidence
- Help identify weaknesses

Once you have stabilized, *then* you stand.

# CHAPTER 17

## SQUATS

# THE BOTTOM POSITION OF THE SQUAT

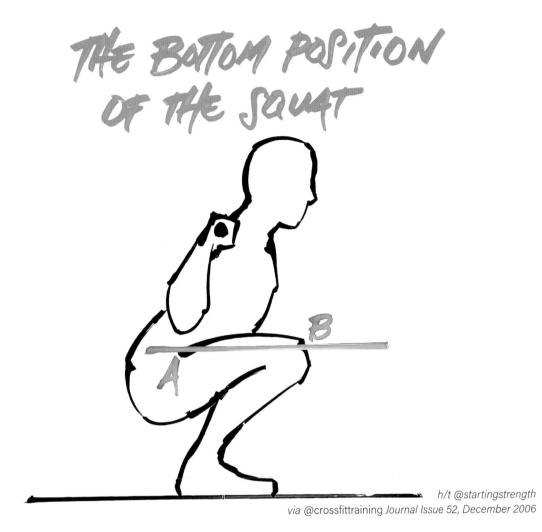

*h/t @startingstrength*
*via @crossfittraining Journal Issue 52, December 2006*

## What does this mean?

The movement standard for the squat involves the athlete starting and finishing in a standing position. A good rep is complete once the athlete stands after squatting to the point the crease of their hip passes below the top of their knee.

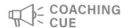
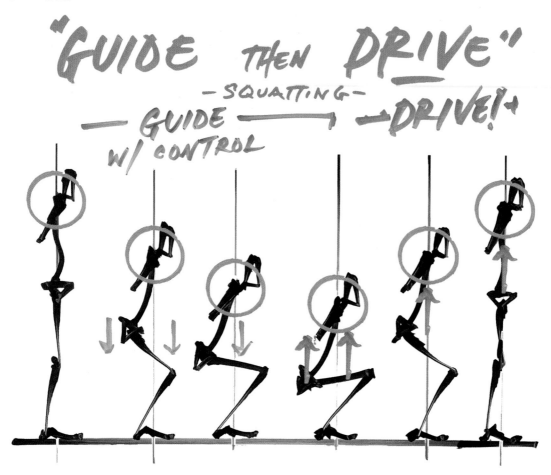

"GUIDE THEN DRIVE"
— SQUATTING —
— GUIDE ———————→ →DRIVE!←
w/ CONTROL

## When?

Squats

## What does this mean?

It's no secret that better positioning leads to more power. During the squat, the less control you have during the descent (eccentric portion), the less power you have on the ascent (concentric portion). As you lower into the squat, think about *guiding* the weight with control. As soon as you reach depth, *drive* it out of the bottom.

## Why is this important?

Maintaining good positioning throughout the transition of the lift provides you with the power to stand up.

# "GLUTES TO BOOTS"
## OLY WL STYLE SQUAT

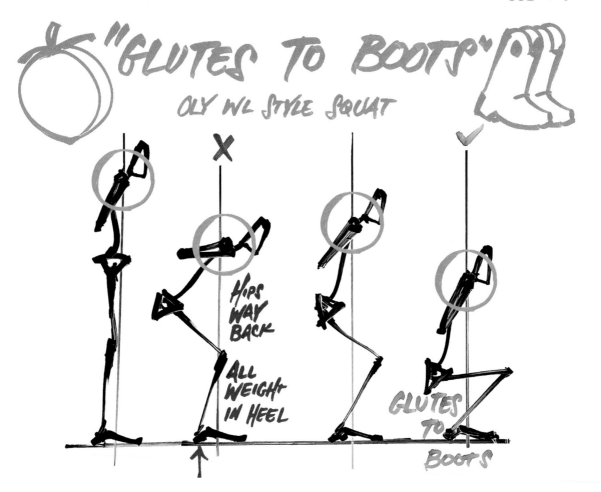

X

HIPS WAY BACK

ALL WEIGHT IN HEEL

✓

GLUTES TO BOOTS

## When?

Olympic weightlifting squat

## What does this mean?

The more upright your torso is, the more efficiently you can support a barbell in the back rack, front rack, or overhead position. By bringing your rear end (glutes) to your heels (boots), you are able to keep the weight over the middle of your foot and your torso in an advantageous position.

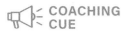
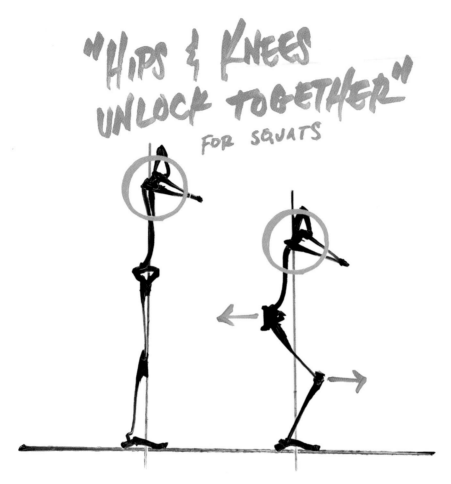

"HIPS & KNEES UNLOCK TOGETHER" FOR SQUATS

## When?
Squatting in weightlifting

## What does this mean?
As you initiate the squat, pressurize your trunk, set the proper arch of your back, and bend your hips and knees at the same time, keeping your torso upright and stacked. Keep even pressure through the tripod of your foot throughout the movement.

## Why is this important?
Bending your hips and knees at the same time during a squat helps you keep a strong and balanced movement pattern.

# "HIPS TO HEELS"
## WHEN SQUATING

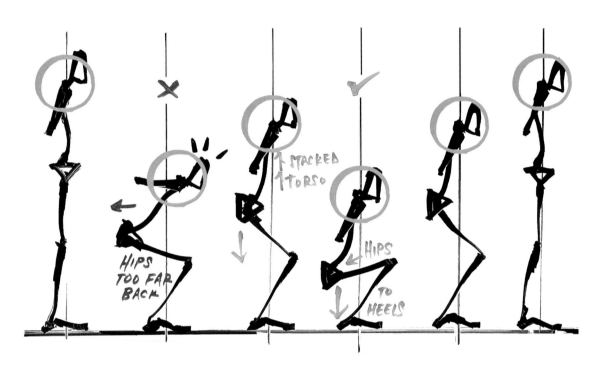

## When?

Olympic weightlifting squat

## What does this mean?

A common error during the squat is sitting back rather than down. Sending the hips back leans the torso forward, resulting in a weaker position, especially when you're holding weight in the front or back rack. Instead, aim to send your hips to your heels when you're descending.

## Why is this important?

Sending your hips to your heels helps keep your torso upright and in a strong, stacked position.

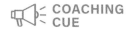
# "IMAGINARY INDO BOARD"
## EQUAL PRESSURE THROUGH BOTH FEET

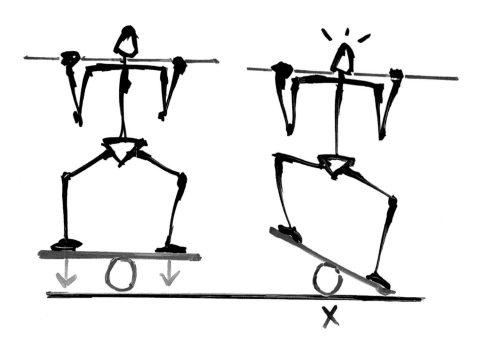

## When?

Applying equal pressure through both feet

## What does this mean?

The INDO BOARD is a simple and effective balance trainer that uses a deck and a roller. When I have an athlete who demonstrates uneven pressure through their feet during squats or deadlifts, I'll suggest they imagine they are on an INDO BOARD. This often helps the athlete apply equal pressure and even up their balance.

# "POCKETS BELOW KNEES"
## — TEACHING THE SQUAT STANDARD —

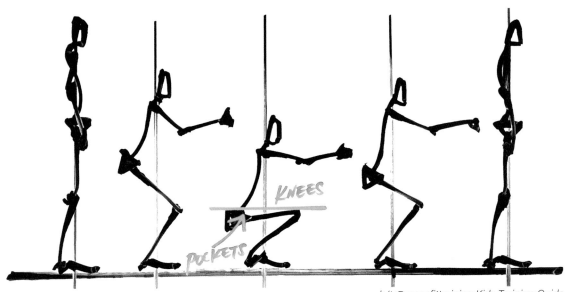

*h/t @crossfittraining Kids Training Guide*

## When?

Teaching the squat standard

## What does this mean?

Some athletes, especially younger ones, might not take much meaning from a cue like "Hip crease below the top of the knee." Another way to say "hip crease" can be "pockets."

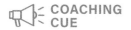

COACHING
CUE

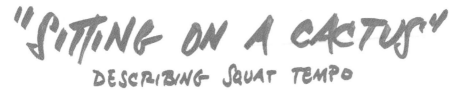

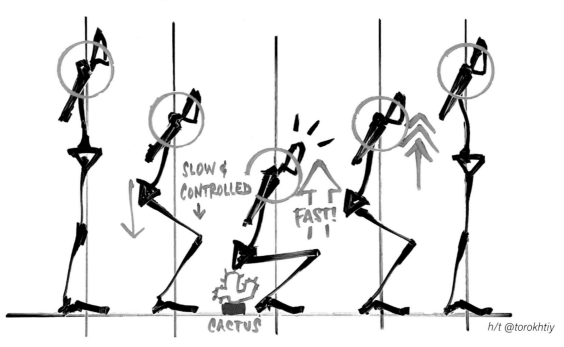

h/t @torokhtiy

## When?

Describing tempo during the squat

## What does this mean?

SLOW ↓ FAST ↑

Squatting with a controlled descent allows for an efficient ascent with optimal control. When you're squatting, imagine your rear end makes contact with a cactus at the bottom of the squat. In that situation, you'd move quickly off the cactus, just as you should drive fast out of the bottom of the squat.

## Why is this important?

Squatting with this tempo will help train your body to create maximum force throughout the concentric portion of the lift.

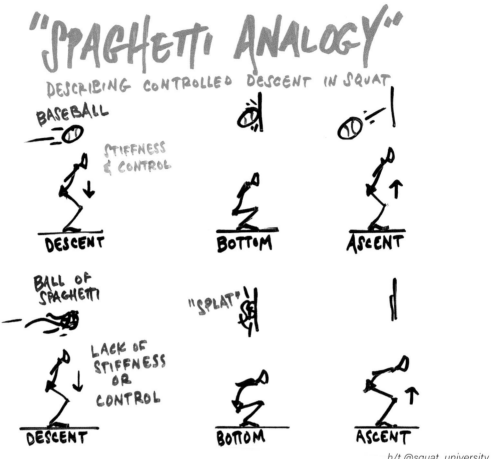

# "SPAGHETTI ANALOGY"

## DESCRIBING CONTROLLED DESCENT IN SQUAT

BASEBALL

STIFFNESS & CONTROL

DESCENT        BOTTOM        ASCENT

BALL OF SPAGHETTI

"SPLAT"

LACK OF STIFFNESS OR CONTROL

DESCENT        BOTTOM        ASCENT

*h/t @squat_university*

## When?

Incorporating diaphragmatic breathing (belly breathing) to brace under load (e.g., heavy squats)

## What does this mean?

Imagine throwing a baseball at a wall. The baseball is constructed of dense rubber and tightly wound yarn, and it's wrapped in stretched leather. When the hard ball hits the wall, the energy from the ball is transferred, and it bounces back.

Now imagine throwing a ball of spaghetti at a wall. Spaghetti is a loose mess of noodles. When a handful of spaghetti hits the wall, there is no energy transfer. Just... splat!

Similarly, when you're back squatting, maintaining a controlled descent with organized muscular engagement allows for efficient ascent with optimal control.

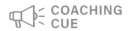

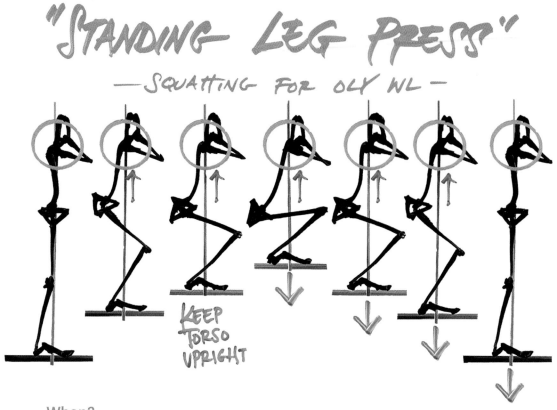

"STANDING LEG PRESS"
— SQUATTING FOR OLY WL —

KEEP TORSO UPRIGHT

## When?

Squatting for Olympic weightlifting

## What does this mean?

Keep your torso as upright as possible as you move through the full range of motion for the squat.

When you're using a leg press machine, your back angle does not change. As you squat, imagine locking your torso into as vertical a position as possible and the floor moving up and down.

# "TRAPEZOID NOT RECTANGLE"
## — HIPS / KNEES / TORSO POSITION —
### DURING SQUAT

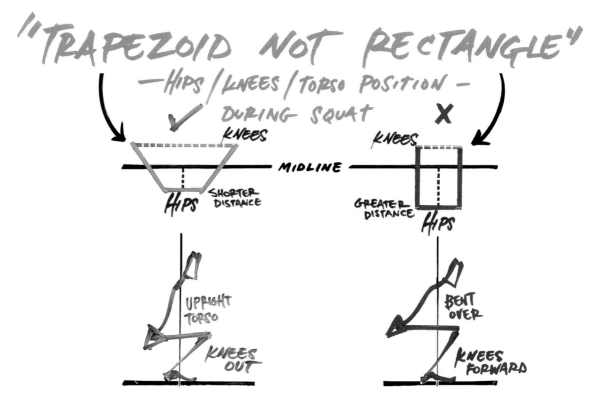

## When?

Knee, hip, and torso position during squat (and dip)

## What does this mean?

From a top-down perspective, your hips and knees should make a trapezoid shape during the squat.

## Why is this important?

A rectangle shape is less efficient because

- Your feet are approximately shoulder width.
- Your toes are pointed forward.
- Your knees track straight forward.

A rectangle shape sends your hips back. If your hips move back, your torso must lean forward to keep the weight over the mid-foot.

A trapezoid shape is more efficient because

- Your feet are approximately shoulder width.
- Your toes are slightly pointed out.
- Your knees track outward in the same direction as your toes throughout movement.

A trapezoid shape allows your hips to stay closer to the midline. The closer your hips are to the midline of your body, the more upright your torso.

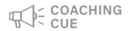
COACHING
CUE

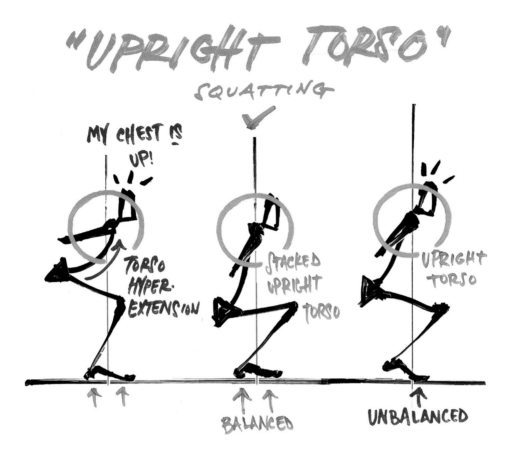

"UPRIGHT TORSO"
SQUATTING ✓

MY CHEST IS UP!

TORSO HYPER. EXTENSION

STACKED UPRIGHT TORSO

UPRIGHT TORSO

BALANCED

UNBALANCED

## When?

Squatting

## What does this mean?

A common cue for the squat is "chest up." Although this may work for many athletes, it does not properly address the errors that keep the athlete from achieving a strong position.

An athlete may fight to keep their chest up, but lose strength through hyperextension of their torso. The torso is most stable for supporting weight (back rack, front rack, overhead) when it is in an upright, stacked position. Equally important is having balanced pressure through the tripod of the foot during the entire movement of the squat.

## Why is this important?

Balanced foot pressure + upright torso = strongest biomechanical position

# "THE ZERCHER SQUAT"

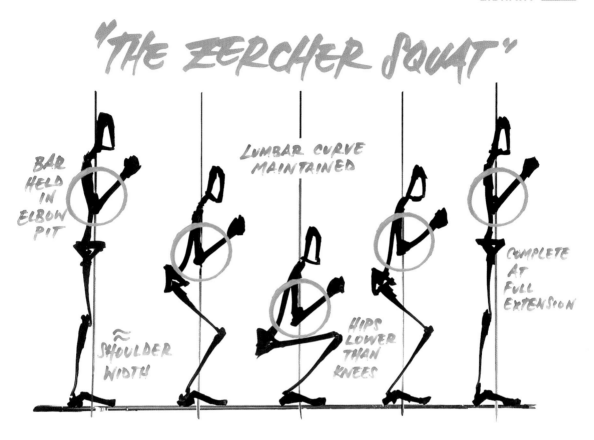

BAR HELD IN ELBOW PIT

LUMBAR CURVE MAINTAINED

SHOULDER WIDTH

HIPS LOWER THAN KNEES

COMPLETE AT FULL EXTENSION

## Points of Performance

### Setup:

- Approximate shoulder-width stance
- Bar resting in the bend of the elbows

### Movement:

- Hips descend back and down.
- Hips descend lower than the knees.
- Maintain lumbar curve.
- Keep heels grounded.
- Keep knee direction in line with toe direction.

The movement is complete at full hip and knee extension.

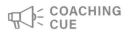

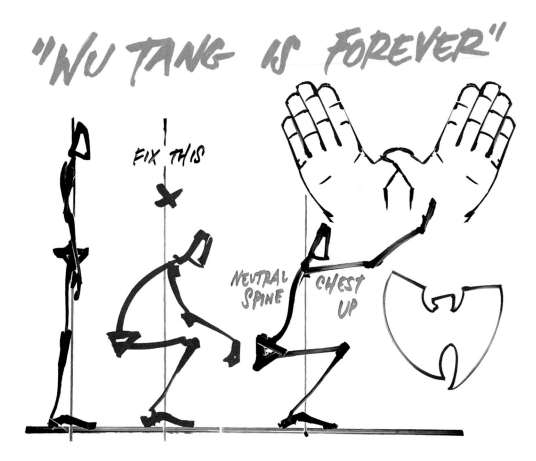

"WU TANG IS FOREVER"

FIX THIS

NEUTRAL SPINE

CHEST UP

## When?

For athletes who tend to bow forward when they air squat.

## What does this mean?

Try standing tall and extending your arms slightly above your head (at about 45°), as if you are holding up the Wu Tang sign. Keep your arms in this position as you move through the full range of movement of your squat.

## Why is this important?

Loss of a neutral spine in a squat puts you in a weak, compromised position. Extending your arms helps keep your chest up and activates muscles in your back, leading to better positioning.

# "BACK INTO THE BAR"
## STANDING UP THE BACK SQUAT

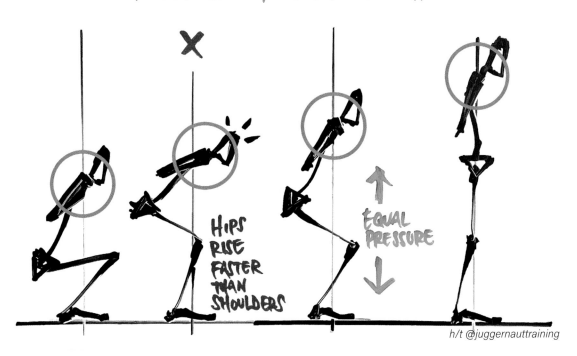

X

HIPS
RISE
FASTER
THAN
SHOULDERS

EQUAL
PRESSURE

h/t @juggernauttraining

## When?

Back squatting, especially if your hips rise quicker than the shoulders

## What does this mean?

Drive your back up into the bar.

## Why is this important?

Efficient movement for the back squat happens when your hips and shoulders rise at the same time. If your hips are moving but your shoulders (where the barbell is) are not, there's a leak of power. Thinking "back into the bar" may help you focus on moving both of these body parts together in unison.

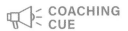

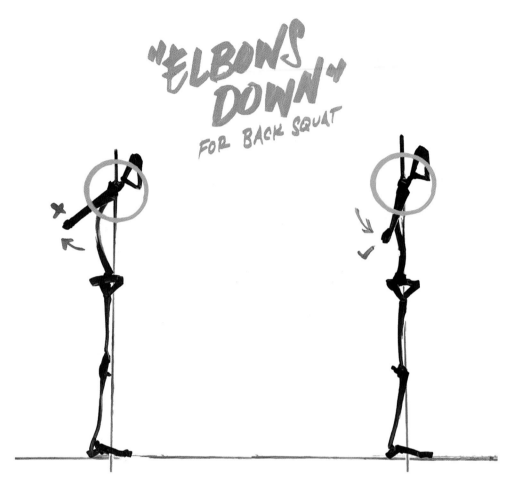

## When?

Back squat

## What does this mean?

Tuck your elbows down toward your midline and next to your torso.

## Why is this important?

Tucking your elbows helps

- Keep your torso in an upright and strong position throughout the movement

- Engage your lats and creates tension through your upper back

- Evenly distribute the weight of the bar perpendicularly, placing more of the stress on your quads and less on your lower back

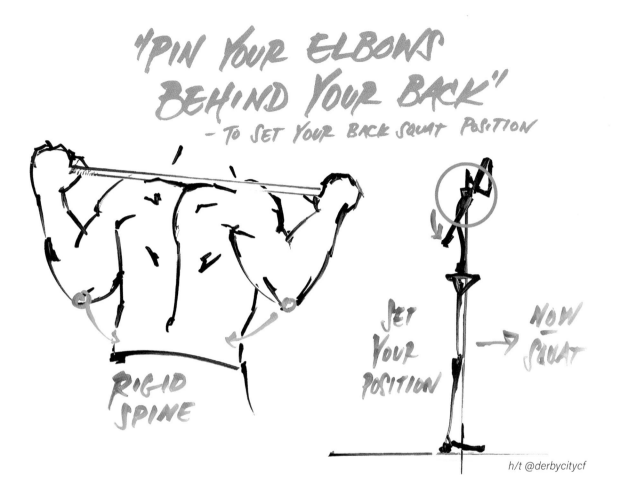

# "PIN YOUR ELBOWS BEHIND YOUR BACK"
## — TO SET YOUR BACK SQUAT POSITION

RIGID SPINE

SET YOUR POSITION

NOW SQUAT

h/t @derbycitycf

## When?

Setting position for back squats

## What does this mean?

Prior to descending during the barbell back squat, aggressively pin your elbows behind your back to engage your traps, delts, and your mighty lats, creating a strong, rigid torso.

## Why is this important?

Pinning your elbows behind your back establishes a solid platform for the bar to rest and allows for an efficient transfer of power from the leg drive into the bar.

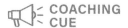

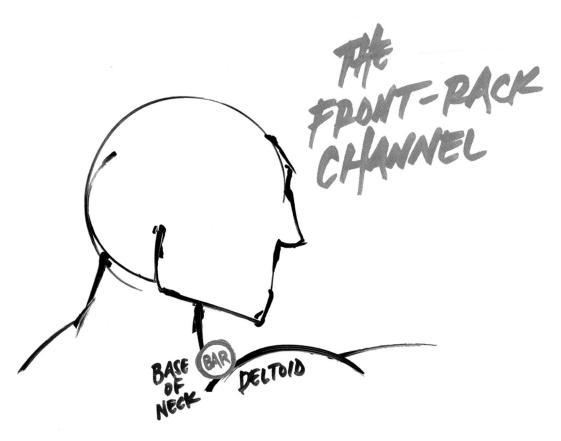

## When?

Front-rack barbell movements

## What does this mean?

In an optimal front-rack position, the barbell sits in the channel between the base of your neck and the rear of your deltoids.

## Why is this important?

This position provides you with a stable shelf that connects the bar with your torso and keeps it close to the midline.

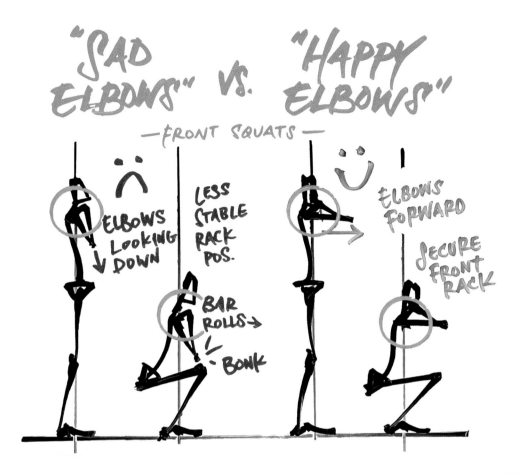

# "SAD ELBOWS" vs. "HAPPY ELBOWS"
## — FRONT SQUATS —

ELBOWS LOOKING DOWN

LESS STABLE RACK POS.

BAR ROLLS →

BONK

ELBOWS FORWARD

SECURE FRONT RACK

## When?

Fronts squats

## What does this mean?

In an optimal front-rack position, the barbell sits in the channel between the base of your neck and the rear of your deltoids. Driving your elbows forward creates a shelf for the bar to sit comfortably on top of your shoulders and chest.

## Why is this important?

Creating this shelf increases the rigidity of your upper back, which helps you maintain an upright trunk position throughout the entire lift.

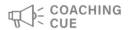
# "MAKE A RIGHT ANGLE"
## —TO FIND OHS GRIP WIDTH—

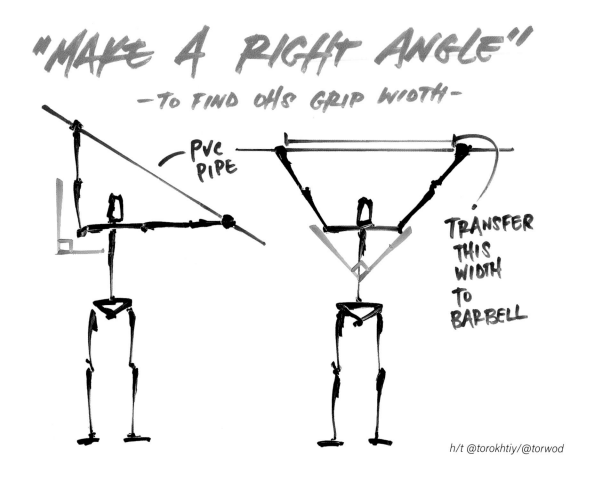

PVC
PIPE

TRANSFER
THIS
WIDTH
TO
BARBELL

h/t @torokhtiy/@torwod

## When?

Finding overhead squat grip width

## What does this mean?

Using a PVC pipe (*not* a barbell), take a wide grip on the bar so that when you extend one arm straight up, that arm and your shoulder make a right angle. Then maintain this width and move your arms so the bar is overhead. Lastly, put down the PVC pipe and pick up the barbell with this same grip width.

*Note:* This drill works for most people but may not work for everyone.

# "MARCH YOUR KNEES"
## — TO FIND OHS/SNATCH GRIP WIDTH —

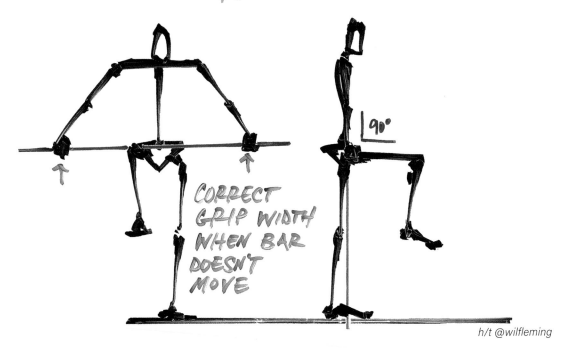

CORRECT
GRIP WIDTH
WHEN BAR
DOESN'T
MOVE

90°

*h/t @wilfleming*

## When?
Establishing snatch/OHS width grip

## How?
Stand, holding the barbell at your waist with your arms long and loose. March your knees high to hip level. You will notice the bar moving up and down from your upper thighs. Widen your grip on the bar until it no longer moves. Once the bar no longer moves, the grip width you have on the bar will work for your snatch and overhead squats.

# CHAPTER ⑱

## STANCE

# "BE A DOG NOT A KITTY CAT"
## LAND w/ A FLAT FOOT FOR CLEAN & SNATCH

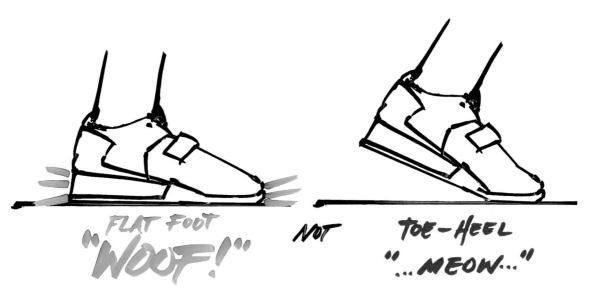

FLAT FOOT
"WOOF!"

NOT

TOE-HEEL
"...MEOW..."

## When?

Landing during the snatch and clean

## What does this mean?

Landing with flat feet = POP = WOOF! (dog)

Landing toe-heel = (no sound) = meow (kitty cat)

## Why is this important?

Landing with flat feet when receiving the snatch and clean provides a firm and vertical connection from the ground up. Landing toe-heel creates horizontal movement, which can lead to instability and imbalance.

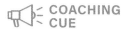

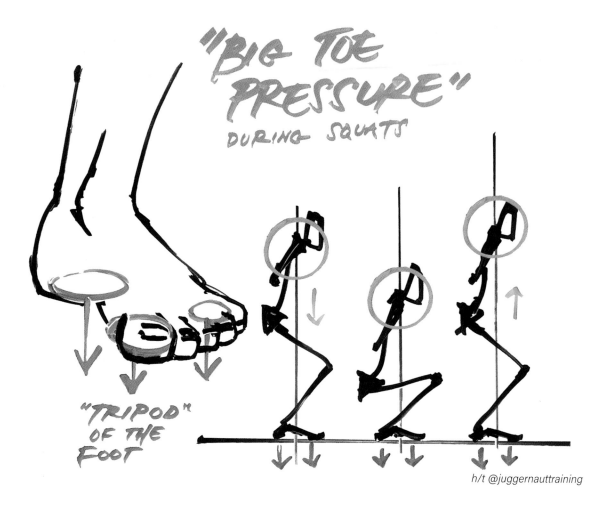

h/t @juggernauttraining

### When?

Squats

### What does this mean?

One of the most common errors for a novice lifter is their heels coming off the ground throughout their squat. Therefore, one of the most common cues for squatting is "heels down." Although this cue may be correct to address that specific issue, it's not always true.

You don't want *all* the weight in the heels. Instead, you want even pressure distributed throughout the big toe, little toe, and heel. Imagining "big toe pressure" tends to solve the issue of not pushing evenly throughout your whole foot.

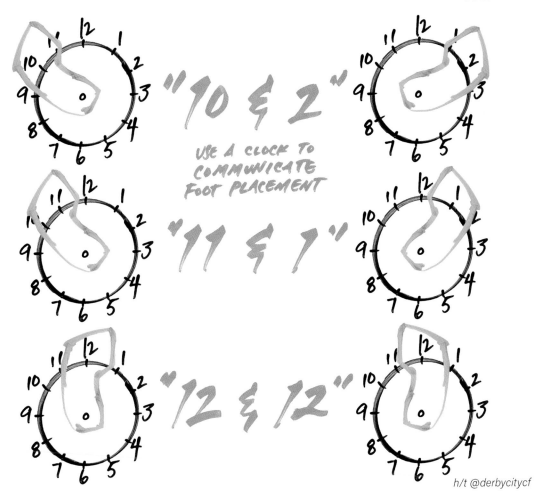

"10 & 2"

USE A CLOCK TO COMMUNICATE FOOT PLACEMENT

"11 & 1"

"12 & 12"

*h/t @derbycitycf*

## When?

Thinking about foot angle placement

## What does this mean?

Imagine your heels in the center of clock faces and direct your toes toward where the numbers would be (based on the angle you want your feet).

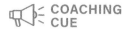
# "EVEN FOOT PRESSURE"
## SQUATTING & DEADLIFTING

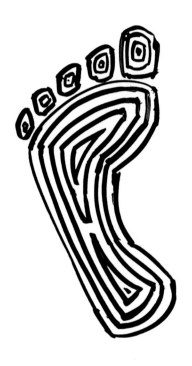
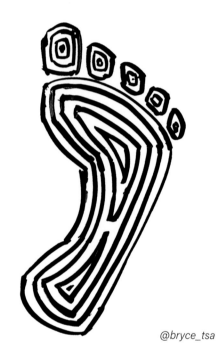

*@bryce_tsa*

### When?

Squatting and deadlifting

### What does this mean?

Quite often, when I see my athletes losing balance throughout a lift or demonstrating a wonky bar path, I simply remind them to slow down and focus on applying even foot pressure: front to back, heel to toe, side to side. Focusing on even foot pressure allows your body to organize itself further up the chain and fixes a lot of subsequent issues.

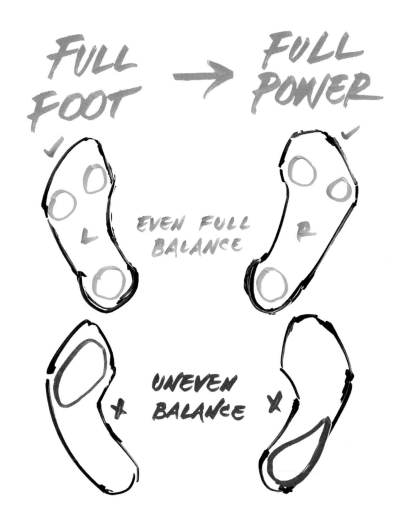

FULL FOOT → FULL POWER

EVEN FULL BALANCE

L   R

UNEVEN BALANCE

## When?

Deadlift, squatting variations, cleans, snatches, and so on

## What does this mean?

When you lift weight, you're pushing the earth away through your feet.

The more connected your feet are to the earth, the more efficiently you can drive the power you generate against the earth.

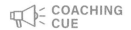
# "HEEL DOWN, TOES DOWN"
## — DURING STANDING LIFTS —

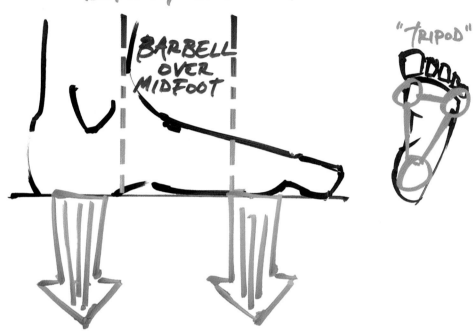

BARBELL OVER MIDFOOT

"TRIPOD"

## When?

Standing lifts

## What does this mean?

During standing lifts, more balance delivers more power. You achieve balance by applying even foot pressure—pressing your foot into the ground with equal pressure through the tripod of your foot (pinky toe, big toe, and heel). In other words, heel down, toes down.

## Why is this important?

Whole-foot balance enables you to keep the bar in the right positions throughout the movement pattern.

In all of the following movements, the bar should stay over the mid-foot region:

- Deadlift
- Sumo deadlift
- Back squat
- Front squat
- Overhead squat

- Snatch
- Hang snatch
- Block snatch
- Power snatch
- Clean
- Hang clean

- Block clean
- Power clean
- Press
- Push press
- Push jerk
- Thruster

# "KNEES IN LINE WITH TOES"

## WHEN SQUATING, LUNGING, DIPPING

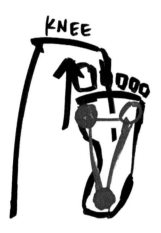
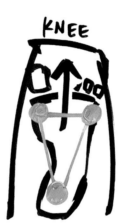
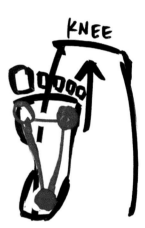

## When?

Squatting, lunging, dipping

## What does this mean?

Connection with your body to the ground happens with your feet. The stronger this connection, the more balanced you become and the more power you can transfer from your body to the ground.

A strong connection occurs with equal pressure through the tripod of your foot. Equal pressure occurs when your knee tracks in line with your toes.

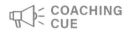
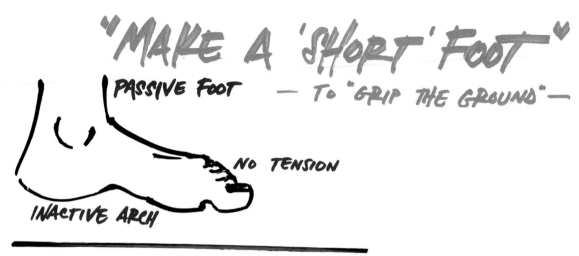

"MAKE A 'SHORT' FOOT"

PASSIVE FOOT — TO "GRIP THE GROUND" —

NO TENSION

INACTIVE ARCH

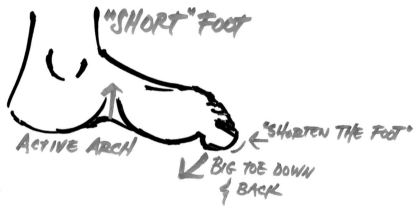

"SHORT" FOOT

ACTIVE ARCH

"SHORTEN THE FOOT"

BIG TOE DOWN & BACK

*h/t @roypumphrey*

## When?

Any standing exercise, especially deadlifts and squats

## What does this mean?

Creating a "short foot" occurs when you grip the ground with your feet. How do you do that? Press your foot into the ground with equal pressure through the tripod of your foot (pinky toe, big toe, and heel).

Further establish this connection by creating torque through your foot, gripping the ground with your toes and slightly rotating your foot externally.

## Why is this important?

Making a short foot engages muscles throughout your legs and creates a stronger connection with the ground.

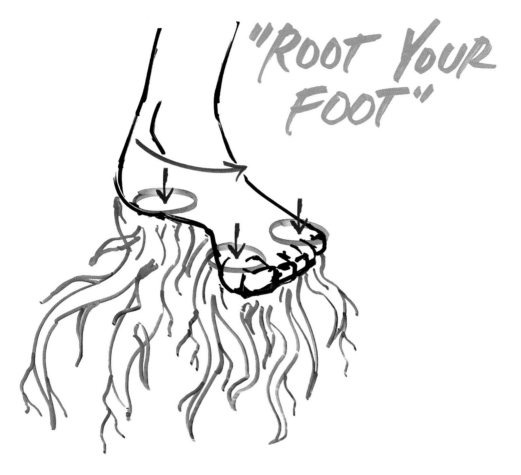

"ROOT YOUR FOOT"

## When?

Any standing exercise, especially deadlifts and squats

## What does this mean?

Press your foot into the ground with equal pressure through the tripod of your foot (pinky toe, big toe, and heel).

Further establish this connection by creating torque through your foot, gripping the ground with your toes, and slightly rotating your foot externally.

Doing so engages muscles throughout your legs and creates a stronger connection with the ground.

This is why footwear is so important. Wear shoes that allow you to feel this connection, or go barefoot.

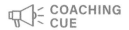
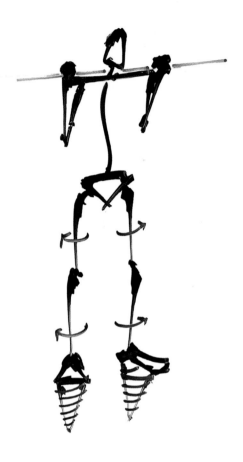

"SCREW YOUR FEET INTO THE GROUND"

*h/t @juggernauttraining*

### When?

Squatting

### What does this mean?

This motion starts as your hips rotate externally and your glutes contract. Your knees rotate out to the side a bit, and your feet move into an arch position. Apply pressure through your big toe to keep your feet from rolling to the side.

### Why is this important?

Gripping the ground correctly sets a firm foundation to perform your best squat.

# "SUCTION CUP YOUR FEET TO THE GROUND."

### – ANY STANDING EXERCISE – ESP. SQUATS

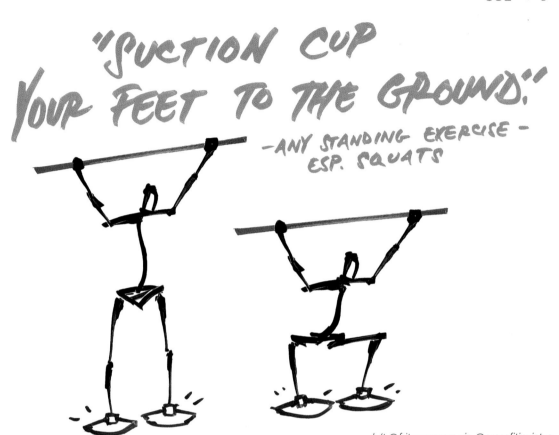

h/t @fritz.program via @crossfitinvictus

## When?

Any standing exercise, especially squats

## What does this mean?

Just as a suction cup grips the surface it's attached to, you should create an active foot and grip the ground with your feet.

## How do you do that?

Press your foot into the ground with equal pressure through the tripod of your foot (pinky toe, big toe, and heel). Further this connection by creating torque through your foot, gripping the ground with your toes, and slightly externally rotating your foot.

## Why is this important?

Gripping the ground with your feet engages muscles throughout your legs, creates a stronger connection with the ground, and improves balance.

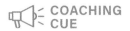

# "WIPE YOUR FEET ON A DOORMAT"

## — FOR HIP-WIDTH STANCE —

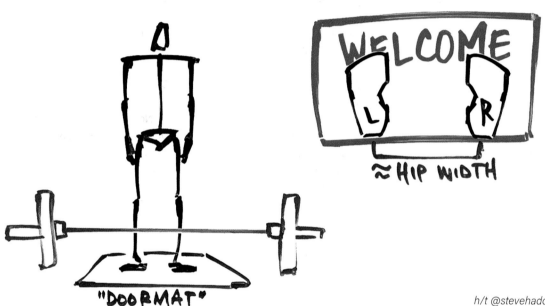

"DOORMAT"

≈ HIP WIDTH

*h/t @stevehadock*

## When?

Taking a hip-width stance, the general stance for pulling, pressing, and jumping movements

## How do you do that?

Act like you're wiping your feet on a door mat and then stand with your feet hip width apart.

# TITLE INDEX